DIGESTIVE DISEASES - RESEARCH AND CLINICAL DEVELOPMENTS

GASTROESOPHAGEAL REFLUX DISEASE (GERD)

CLINICAL CHARACTERISTICS, MANAGEMENT AND LONG-TERM OUTCOMES

DIGESTIVE DISEASES - RESEARCH AND CLINICAL DEVELOPMENTS

Additional books in this series can be found on Nova's website under the Series tab.

Additional e-books in this series can be found on Nova's website under the e-book tab.

DIGESTIVE DISEASES - RESEARCH AND CLINICAL DEVELOPMENTS

GASTROESOPHAGEAL REFLUX DISEASE (GERD)

CLINICAL CHARACTERISTICS, MANAGEMENT AND LONG-TERM OUTCOMES

LARRY P. CORNETT
EDITOR

NOVA BIOMEDICAL
New York

Library of Congress Cataloging-in-Publication Data

ISBN: 978-1-63484-125-2

Library of Congress Control Number: 2015955198

Published by Nova Science Publishers, Inc. † New York

CONTENTS

PREFACE

Gastroesophageal reflux disease (GERD) is a common disorder affecting approximately more than 10% of the population. GERD is highly heterogeneous in terms of varied manifestations, test findings and treatment responsiveness. The invasive treatment options for GERD have now greatly expanded from just the Nissen Fundoplication to various other options such as other minimally invasive options like the Lower Esophageal augmentation with a magnetic device, and multiple endoscopic options like Radiofrequency ablation, Trans-oral incisionless fundoplication (TIF) etc. Treatment options require an understanding of the patho-physiology of GERD, which is discussed in chapter one of this book. Chapter two studies the clinical practices for extra-esophageal reflux and explores the outcomes. Chapter three reviews extraesophageal reflux and sleep microarchitecture disturbance and excessive daytime sleepiness. Chapter four discusses osteopathic manipulative therapy. The final chapter provides updated research on the surgical treatment options for GERD and their long-term outcomes.

Chapter 1 - Gastro Esophageal Reflux Disease (GERD) has a complex patho-physiology. The invasive treatment options for GERD have now greatly expanded from just the Nissen Fundoplication to various other options such as other minimally invasive options like the Lower Esophageal augmentation with a magnetic device, and multiple endoscopic options like Radiofrequency ablation, Trans-oral incisionless fundoplication (TIF) etc. These treatment options have their specific role and should be individualized to patients, which requires understanding of the patho-physiology of GERD.

There are a lot of proposed theories and concepts regarding the patho-physiology of GERD. Stein and coworkers gave us the concept of the plumbing circuit where the esophagus functions as antegrade pump, the Lower esophageal sphincter (LES) as a valve, and stomach as a reservoir. Problems with any component of the circuit (either poor esophageal motility or a dysfunctional LES or delayed gastric emptying) can lead to GERD.

Another cause of reflux is a hypotensive Lower esophageal sphincter (LES). Transient inappropriate LES relaxations (TLESR) (relaxation in the absence of swallowing) are also a relatively newer concept in the causation of reflux. Prolonged or more frequent TLESRs have been investigated as a cause of reflux. Apart from the LES itself the diaphragmatic crura, and the phreno-esophageal ligament, which help form the angle of His also have a role in preventing reflux. A hiatal hernia also contributes to reflux as proximal migration of the LES may result in loss of its abdominal high-pressure zone (HPZ). Herein the authors will discuss some of these mechanisms in the patho-physiology of GERD.

Chapter 2 - Gastroesophageal reflux disease (GERD) is a common disorder affecting more than 10% of the population. GERD is highly heterogeneous in terms of varied manifestations, test findings and treatment responsiveness. Acid regurgitation and heartburn are known as typical symptoms of GERD. However, GERD can often represented as atypical symptom of chest pain, as well as extraesophageal symptoms such as chough and asthma. Extraesophageal reflux requires sufficient awareness, understanding and evaluation. Multidisciplinary integrated treatment from medical to surgical strategy should be followed in the management of extraesophageal symptoms, according to the severity, reflux character, therapy responsiveness of individual extraesophageal symptoms.

Chapter 3 - Gastroesophageal Reflux (GER) has a high prevalence. It should be differentiated between the symptomatic reflux and the so called "silent" Extraesophageal Reflux (EER) with dominant ENT-symptoms. Additionally, it should be noticed that there is a high coincidence with Obstructive Sleep Apnea (OSA).

A pilot study shows that the core symptom of OSA Excessive Daytime Sleepiness (EDS) is also similarly common in EER. The background for this is the sleep microstructure particularly in view of the Cyclic Alternating Pattern (CAP) with the different subtypes. Reflux episodes are not linked to respiratory events.

Reflux events are associated with high arousal activity and simultaneously with increased variability of Heart Frequency (HF) and Pulse-Transit-Time (PTT) – similar to respiratory induced arousals. The usual classification of sleep structure is not useful with regard to the EDS.

With respect to the importance of persistent daytime sleepiness in effective nocturnal ventilated OSA-patients, further appropriate investigations are mandatory.

Chapter 4 - Gastroesophageal reflux disease (GERD) is a chronic condition that affects a growing number of subjects, and is one of the most prevalent diseases in clinical practice.In the US, it has been estimated that GERD has the highest annual direct costs of all gastrointestinal diseases, at $9.3 billion.

Heartburn is the most predominant esophageal symptom of GERD, while bronchospasm and chronic cough are the most common extraesophageal symptoms.Gastroesophageal reflux disease compromises patient quality of life by requiring modification of the patients' eating habits.The resulting changes in sleep patterns, as well as other various recurrent or lasting long-term symptoms, may limit daily activities.

The digestive system presents a complex anatomic and physiologic relationship, starting at the cranial base with the attachments of the esophagus via pharyngeal tubercle, down to the hyoid bone, the sixth cervical vertebra (C6), the diaphragm and the lesser omentum; also the liver, spleen, kidney and the greater omentum for the stomach.

The esophagogastric junction (EGJ) is a complex valvular structure that prevents reflux, is composed of the intrinsic lower esophageal sphincter (LES), is situated within the diaphragmatic hiatus, and is surrounded by the crural diaphragm (CD), which provides additional sphincteric compression. It is the main barrier against gastroesophageal reflux, and its function has been attributed to intrinsic LES pressure, extrinsic compression of the LES by the CD, the intraabdominal location of the LES, integrity of the phrenoesophageal ligament, and maintenance of the acute angle between the esophagus and stomach, promoting a "flap valve" function.

Vagal preganglionic efferents innervate the LES smooth muscle, both excitatory and inhibitory innervation. Sympathetic efferents from the spinal segments T6 through T10 are likely primarily nociceptive and potential modulators of LES relaxation induced by the vagus nerve. Thus, the vagus nerve is the prime mediator of LES reflexes.

Osteopathic medicine relies on manual contact for diagnosis and treatment, based on the structural and functional integrity of the body and its intrinsic capacity for self-healing. Osteopathic practitioners use a wide variety of manual techniques to improve physiological function and/or support homeostasis that has been altered by somatic dysfunction, i.e., impaired or altered function of related components of the somatic system; skeletal, arthrodial and myofascial structures; and related vascular, lymphatic, and neural elements.

Dysfunctions at the cranial base, lower cervical vertebrae, thoracic inlet, a compromised CD function, and altered distensibility of the hiatal canal, dysfunctions of the diaphragm, liver and stomach could be considered structural factors leading to GERD. Conversely, dysfunctions of the cranial base and the thoracic inlet could affect the vagus nerve, cervical (C3-C4) dysfunctions could affect the phrenic nerve and alter the movement of the diaphragm and EGJ, and thoracic (between T6-T10) dysfunctions could affect the sympathetic innervation of the LES.

Therefore, a detailed assessment of all aspects related to the LES function, directly or not, would provide useful data to draw an appropriate osteopathic manipulative approach, whether addressed to the innervation zones or to the anatomical structures directly related to the LES.

Chapter 5 - Gastroesophageal reflux disease (GERD) is a very frequent pathology in developed countries. After failure of initial medical treatment, mainly based on Proton Pump Inhibitors (PPI), surgery is indicated. The goal of antireflux operation is to achieve control of the symptoms with minimum risk and without adding any long-term side effects to the patient undergoing the procedure. Laparoscopic approach has become the elective approach for the surgical treatment of GERD in the last decade. Compared with conventional surgery, laparoscopy presents lower complication and mortality rates, and a shorter hospital stay. There is a great controversy about the fundoplication technique of choice. Nissen funcoplication seems to be the better antireflux technique for some authors, presenting the smaller recurrence rate. However, Nissen fundoplication is also associated with higher incidence of dysphagia, that may reach up to 20% of the cases.

Outcome data beyond 10 years describe good-to-excellent outcomes in most patients. The durability of fundoplication has been documented with more than 90% of patients satisfied after 10 years, without recurrence of reflux symptoms or appearance of dysphagia.

In this chapter the authors will review the actual evidence about all these issues.

In: Gastroesophageal Reflux Disease (GERD) ISBN: 978-1-63484-125-2
Editor: Larry P. Cornett

Chapter 1

PATHO-PHYSIOLOGY OF GASTRO ESOPHAGEAL REFLUX DISEASE

Vikas Singhal, MRCS (Glasgow)
Consultant- Minimal Access, GI and Bariatric Surgery,
Jaypee Hospital, Noida, India

ABSTRACT

Gastro Esophageal Reflux Disease (GERD) has a complex patho-physiology. The invasive treatment options for GERD have now greatly expanded from just the Nissen Fundoplication to various other options such as other minimally invasive options like the Lower Esophageal augmentation with a magnetic device, and multiple endoscopic options like Radiofrequency ablation, Trans-oral incisionless fundoplication (TIF) etc. These treatment options have their specific role and should be individualized to patients, which requires understanding of the patho-physiology of GERD.

There are a lot of proposed theories and concepts regarding the patho-physiology of GERD. Stein and coworkers gave us the concept of the plumbing circuit where the esophagus functions as antegrade pump, the Lower esophageal sphincter (LES) as a valve, and stomach as a reservoir. Problems with any component of the circuit (either poor esophageal motility or a dysfunctional LES or delayed gastric emptying) can lead to GERD.

Another cause of reflux is a hypotensive Lower esophageal sphincter (LES). Transient inappropriate LES relaxations (TLESR) (relaxation in the absence of swallowing) are also a relatively newer concept in the causation of reflux. Prolonged or more frequent TLESRs have been investigated as a cause of reflux. Apart from the LES itself the diaphragmatic crura, and the phreno-esophageal ligament, which help form the angle of His also have a role in preventing reflux. A hiatal hernia also contributes to reflux as proximal migration of the LES may result in loss of its abdominal high-pressure zone (HPZ). Herein we will discuss some of these mechanisms in the patho-physiology of GERD.

Patho-Physiology of Gastro Esophageal Reflux Disease

Gastro Esophageal Reflux Disease (GERD) has a complex patho-physiology. With multiple treatment options now available for GERD ranging from medication to endoscopic treatment to surgical treatment understanding the pathophysiology of GERD has become even more important as to be able to appropriately counsel patients we need to understand which method would be more suitable for the particular patient. To understand the patho-physiology of GERD we first need to understand the various mechanisms that come into play to prevent reflux. There are varying roles of various structures starting from the Upper esophageal sphincter (UES), then the esophageal swallowing (peristaltic) mechanism, then the Lower esophageal sphincter (LES) which is supported from the outside by the diaphragm and its attachments and finally the gastric emptying. Stein and coworkers put this together and simplified it to give us the concept of the plumbing circuit where the esophagus functions as an antegrade pump, the Lower esophageal sphincter (LES) as a valve, and the stomach as a reservoir [1]. Problems with any component of the circuit either poor esophageal motility or a dysfunctional LES or delayed gastric emptying can lead to GERD. From a medical or surgical standpoint, it is extremely important to identify which of these components is defective so that effective therapy can be applied. We will first describe these components separately and then put them together.

The Upper Esophageal Sphincter (UES)

The upper esophageal sphincter is formed by the cervical esophagus, the cricopharyngeus muscle, and inferior pharyngeal constrictor, but primarily the cricopharyngeus. The main functions of the UES are to prevent esophageal air insufflation during inspiration, and to prevent esophagopharyngeal/laryngeal reflux during esophageal peristalsis. Initially the role of UES in preventing GERD was thought to be less significant and its length was underestimated. Hernandez et al. studied the UES and correlated the Manometric and Ultrasound findings and found that manometrically, the UES-HPZ had a median length of 4.0 cm (range 3.0-4.5 cm) [2]. A C-shaped muscle, believed to represent the cricopharyngeus muscle, was observed for a median length of 3.5 cm (range 2.0-4.0 cm).

A recent study by Babaei et al. demonstrated that the UES may indeed have a significant role in preventing Supra-esophageal reflux disease (SERD) [3]. In their study they used High Resolution Manometry (HRM) with impedance to assess simulated response of the UES and esophageal peristalsis to slow and rapid infusion of air and liquid. They found that a significantly smaller proportion of patients with SERD had UES contractile reflexes in response to slow esophageal infusion of acid than controls or patients with GERD. Only patients with SERD had abnormal UES relaxation responses to rapid distension with saline.

A dysfunctional UES may indeed contribute significantly to Laryngo-esophageal reflux (LER).

Esophageal Peristalsis

Esophageal peristaltic mechanisms are responsible for clearing the esophagus of its volume, saliva, acid and refluxate. Esophageal peristalsis results from sequential contraction of the circular muscle that pushes the ingested food bolus toward the stomach. Esophageal longitudinal muscle may also play a role in peristalsis. The peristalsis in response to swallowing is called primary peristalsis, and the subsequent peristaltic wave due to esophageal distention is called secondary peristalsis.

Some patients with reflux disease, particularly those with severe esophagitis, exhibit impaired esophageal responses to reflux [4, 5]. Kahrilas et al. demonstrated in their study that degree of peristaltic dysfunction correlated with the severity of esophagitis, occurring in 25% of patients with mild esophagitis and 48% of patients with severe esophagitis [6].

Sun et al. compared manometric analyses in patients with reflux esophagitis to those in patients with Non-erosive disease (NERD) and found that peristaltic contraction amplitude of distal esophageal body and rate of effective peristaltic contraction of distal esophageal body were significantly lower in the reflux esophagitis group than in the NERD group [7]. It may not be possible to determine in some cases what came first, whether over time Gastro Esophageal reflux (GER) led to dysfunctional esophageal peristalsis, rather than dysfunctional peristalsis leading to GER.

It is likely that reduced esophageal peristalsis not only prolongs acid clearance but also influences the proximal extent of the refluxate within the esophageal body as shown by HRM with impedance testing.

The Esophago-Gastric Junction

Apart from the Lower Esophageal Sphincter (LES) itself there are two other anatomical structures that contribute to preventing reflux at the esophago-gastric junction which are the diaphragmatic crura, and the phreno-esophageal ligament.

The LES is defined by manometry as a zone of elevated intraluminal pressure at the esophagogastric junction. It is a 3-4 cm segment of contracted circular smooth muscle at the distal end of the esophagus, the resting tone of which varies from 10 mm Hg to 35 mm Hg. Acid reflux occurs when an increase in intra-abdominal pressure exceeds the hypotensive LES pressure. The right crus of the diaphragm forms a sling like mechanism and contributes to the Angle of His. The angle of His is the acute angle created between the esophagus and the gastric cardia.

For proper LES function, the Esophago-gastric junction must be located in the abdomen so that the diaphragmatic crura can assist the action of the LES, thus functioning as an extrinsic sphincter.

Bombeck et al. way back in 1966 in an autopsy study proved that the phrenoesophageal ligament indeed existed and had a role in supporting the LES in preventing GER [8]. It has been proposed that the ligament has two layers, arising from the endothoracic fascia and a thicker circumferential continuation of the endoabdominal (transversalis) fascia. If this mechanism is defective a hiatus hernia may result.

A hiatal hernia may contribute to reflux as proximal migration of the LES may result in loss of its abdominal high-pressure zone (HPZ), or the length of the HPZ may decrease [9]. Also the crural mechanisms will not be effective in preventing reflux [10]. A significant association has been demonstrated with an irreducible hiatus hernia on Barium swallow study and esophagitis [11].

Hence reduction of the hiatal hernia with re-establishing the intra-abdominal length of the esophagus with proper crural closure, apart from a fundic wrap are key components to surgical correction of GERD.

TRANSIENT LOWER ESOPHAGEAL SPHINCTER RELAXATIONS (TLESRS)

There occur a normal number of episodes of transient relaxation of the LES (relaxation in the absence of swallowing). These transient lower esophageal sphincter relaxations (TLESRs) are possibly vagally mediated reflxes and serve to vent the stomach. TLESRs are now thought to be the most common mechanism of the physiologic reflux episodes noted on pH study. It has also been hypothesized that prolonged or more frequents TLESRs may be the dominant cause of reflux disease in a subset of patients with GERD. Pauwels et al. studied the relationship between changes in intragastric pressure and TLESRs [12]. They found a clear negative correlation between change in intra-gastric pressure and the number of TLESRs, irrespective of whether they were associated with reflux or not, both in GERD patients and in healthy subjects. These results suggest that TLESRs and GA are closely linked, probably through activation of mechanoreceptors involved in triggering of TLESRs.

Gastric Emptying

Delayed gastric emptying as in pregnancy, diabetic patients etc may contribute to GERD however its role does not seem significant. Patient whose symptoms include nausea or vomiting may be suffering from delayed gastric emptying and may require a gastric emptying study before anti-reflux surgery.

Mucosal Defense Mechanisms

The normal esophageal mucosa defense mechanisms may be overcome by prolonged exposure of the mucosa to a $pH < 4$ that may lead to severe and complicated esophagitis. The defence mechanisms are made up of pre-epithelial, epithelial integrity and other barriers such as the membrane potential etc.

The role of the mucosal barrier has been debated, Szczesniak et al. found in their research that the acid-related sensitization is greater in gastroesophageal reflux disease than in controls and may influence in part symptom perception in this population but this was independent of mucosal inflammation [13].

Obesity Related GERD

A chronically increased intragastric pressure and increased frequency of transient LES relaxations (TLESRs) are thought to play the major role in obesity related GERD.

For morbidly obese patients with Body Mass Index (BMI) more than 40 bariatric surgery has been recommended as a treatment for GERD since the contribution of obesity to GERD is so significant that weight loss becomes paramount in treating the GERD.

Non-Acid Reflux Disease (NARD)

A newer line of investigation is the realization that not reflux is acid. Other components of the refluxate such as bile acids, pepsin, gas etc apart from hypersensitivity to the volume of reflux itself have all been thought to contribute to reflux disease, especially reflux with atypical symptoms and that non-responsive to proton pump inhibitors.

Non-Erosive Reflux Disease (NERD)

Patients who have typical GER symptoms but absence of mucosal changes on upper endoscopy are classified as having NERD. Patients with NERD may not have typical pathologic reflux demonstrated on 24-hour pH study. In such patients factors such as visceral hypersensitivity or more proximal reflux of acid or nonacid material may be important.

Acid and inflammatory mediators may gain access to sensory pathways and produce symptoms either by a direct action on the nerves or by producing abnormal muscle contraction.

CONCLUSION

GERD has a complex pathophysiology and the cause of GERD is different in different patients. With various treatments now available for GERD, and availability of HRM with impedance testing, it is important to understand the pathophysiology of GERD in an individual so that appropriate treatment recommendation can be made.

REFERENCES

[1] Stein HJ, DeMeester TR. Outpatient physiologic testing and surgical management of foregut motility disorders. *Curr Probl Surg* [Internet]. 1992 Jul [cited 2014 Nov 9];29(7):413–555. Available from: http://www.ncbi.nlm.nih.gov/pubmed/1606845.

[2] Hernandez L V, Dua KS, Surapaneni SN, Rittman T, Shaker R. Anatomic-manometric correlation of the upper esophageal sphincter: a concurrent US and manometry study. *Gastrointest Endosc.* 2010;42(2):157–62.

[3] Babaei A, Venu M, Naini SR, Gonzaga J, Lang I, Massey B, et al. Impaired Upper Esophageal Sphincter Reflexes in Patients With Supraesophageal Reflux Disease. *Gastroenterology* [Internet]. 2015 Jul 17 [cited 2015 Oct 4]; Available from: http://www.ncbi.nlm.nih.gov/pubmed/26188682

[4] Holloway RH. Esophageal body motor response to reflux events: *Am J Med* [Internet]. 2000 Mar 6 [cited 2015 Oct 4];108(4):20–6. Available from: http://europepmc.org/abstract/med/10718447.

[5] Aben-Athar CG, Dantas RO. Primary and secondary esophageal contractions in patients with gastroesophageal reflux disease. *Braz j med biol res* [Internet]. [cited 2015 Oct 4];39(8):1027–31. Available from: http://www.scielo.br/scielo.php?script=sci_arttext&pid=S0100-879X2006000800005.

[6] Kahrilas PJ, Dodds WJ, Hogan WJ, Kern M, Arndorfer RC, Reece A. Esophageal peristaltic dysfunction in peptic esophagitis. *Gastroenterology* [Internet]. 1986 Oct [cited 2015 Oct 4];91(4):897–904. Available from: http://www.ncbi.nlm.nih.gov/pubmed/3743966.

[7] Sun X, Ke M, Wang Z, Fang X. [Characteristics of esophageal motility in patients with non-erosive reflux disease and reflux esophagitis].

Zhonghua Yi Xue Za Zhi [Internet]. 2014 Jun 10 [cited 2015 Oct 4];94(22):1718–21. Available from: http://www.ncbi.nlm.nih.gov/pubmed/25151902.

[8] Bombeck CT, Dillard DH, Nyhus LM. Muscular anatomy of the gastroesophageal junction and role of phrenoesophageal ligament; autopsy study of sphincter mechanism. *Ann Surg* [Internet]. 1966 Oct [cited 2015 Oct 4];164(4):643–54. Available from: http://www.pubmedcentral.nih.gov/articlerender.fcgi?artid=1477293&tool=pmcentrez&rendertype=abstract.

[9] Mittal RK, Lange RC, McCallum RW. Identification and mechanism of delayed esophageal acid clearance in subjects with hiatus hernia. *Gastroenterology* [Internet]. 1987 Jan [cited 2015 Aug 28];92(1):130–5. Available from: http://www.ncbi.nlm.nih.gov/pubmed/3781181.

[10] Kahrilas PJ, Lin S, Chen J, Manka M. The effect of hiatus hernia on gastro-oesophageal junction pressure. *Gut* [Internet]. 1999 Apr [cited 2015 Oct 4];44(4):476–82. Available from: http://www.pubmedcentral.nih.gov/articlerender.fcgi?artid=1727465&tool=pmcentrez&rendertype=abstract.

[11] Mattioli S, D'Ovidio F, Pilotti V, Di Simone MP, Lugaresi ML, Bassi F, et al. Hiatus hernia and intrathoracic migration *of esophagogastric junction in gastroesophageal reflux disease. Dig* Dis Sci [Internet]. 2003 Sep [cited 2015 Oct 4];48(9):1823–31. Available from: http://www.ncbi.nlm.nih.gov/pubmed/14561009.

[12] Pauwels A, Altan E, Tack J. The gastric accommodation response to meal intake determines the occurrence of transient lower esophageal sphincter relaxations and reflux events in patients with gastro-esophageal reflux disease. *Neurogastroenterol Motil* [Internet]. 2014 Apr [cited 2015 Oct 7];26(4):581–8. Available from: http://www.ncbi.nlm.nih.gov/pubmed/24533836.

[13] Szczesniak MM, Fuentealba SE, Cook IJ. Acid Sensitization of Esophageal Mucosal Afferents. *Clin J Pain* [Internet]. 2013 Jan [cited 2015 Oct 4];29(1):70–7. Available from: http://www.ncbi.nlm.nih.gov/pubmed/22330131.

In: Gastroesophageal Reflux Disease (GERD) ISBN: 978-1-63484-125-2
Editor: Larry P. Cornett

Chapter 2

CLINICAL PRACTICE FOR EXTRA-ESOPHAGEAL REFLUX AND THE OUTCOME

Zhi-Wei Hu[1], MD, Ji-Min Wu[1], MD and Zhong-Gao Wang[1,2,*], MD, FACS.

[1]Gastroesophageal Reflux Disease Department,
The Second Artillery General Hospital PLA, Beijing, China
[2]Xuanwu Hospital of Capital Medical University, Beijing, China

ABSTRACT

Gastroesophageal reflux disease (GERD) is a common disorder affecting more than 10% of the population. GERD is highly heterogeneous in terms of varied manifestations, test findings and treatment responsiveness. Acid regurgitation and heartburn are known as typical symptoms of GERD. However, GERD can often represented as atypical symptom of chest pain, as well as extraesophageal symptoms such as chough and asthma. Extraesophageal reflux requires sufficient awareness, understanding and evaluation. Multidisciplinary integrated treatment from medical to surgical strategy should be followed in the management of extraesophageal symptoms, according to the severity,

* Correspondence: Wang Zhong-Gao, MD, FACS, Gastroesophageal Reflux Disease Department, the Second Artillery General Hospital PLA, No. 16 Xinwai Street, Xicheng district, Beijing 100088, China. E-mail: zhonggaowang@126.com. Telephone: +86-10-62015718 Fax: +86-10-62015718.

reflux character, therapy responsiveness of individual extraesophageal symptoms.

Keywords: Gastroesophageal reflux disease, extraesophageal reflux, reflux monitoring, proton pump inhibitor, fundoplication, radiofrequency procedure

1. Prevalence of GERD and Extraesophageal Reflux

The prevalence of GERD is estimated more than 10% worldwide and has geographic variation, as estimated 18.1%-27.8% in North America, 8.8%-25.9% in Europe, 2.5%-7.8% in East Asia, 8.7%-33.1% in the Middle East, 11.6% in Australia and 23.0% in South America [1]. About one-third of patients with GERD have frequent and/or severe reflux symptoms. The increasing symptom frequency and severity both increased the burden of disease to a similar extent [2].

However, the overall prevalence of extraesophageal reflux is still unclear and not easy to identify.

High prevalence of extraesophageal symptoms have been found in Korean GERD patients with typical heartburn and regurgitation. globus 51.8%, cough 32.0%, hoarseness 24.2% and wheezing 17.3% [3]. Patients with severe GERD had significantly higher laryngopharyngeal reflux scores compared with mild moderate or inactive disease ones [4]. laryngopharyngeal reflux symptoms may also be influenced significantly by the presence of gastroesophageal reflux [5]. For asthmatic patients, the prevalence of GERD symptoms, abnormal esophageal pH, esophagitis and hiatus hernia was 59.2%, 50.9%, 37.3% and 51.2%, respectively. The average prevalence of asthma in individuals with GERD was 4.6%, whereas in controls it was 3.9% [6]. Pediatricians found that GERD is highly prevalent in children with asthma, as estimates as high as 80%, but nearly half of the children are asymptomatic risks [7].

Gastroesophageal reflux (GER) was also estimated to be associated with 21%-41% cases of chronic cough [8]. The prevalence of chronic rhinosinusitis among patients with GERD was significantly higher than that of the background population (20.7% VS 8.5%) [9]. Pathological extraesophageal reflux in the supine and upright position were found to be as high as 50% and

97% in patients with chronic rhinosinusitis with nasal polyps and simultaneous bronchial asthma by oropharyngeal pH monitoring [10]. The prevalence of GER was significantly higher in patients with COPD than in those without (RR = 13.06; 95% CI: 3.64-46.87; $p < 0.001$). GER was clearly identified as a risk factor for COPD exacerbations (RR = 7.57; 95% CI: 3.84-14.94), with an increased mean number of exacerbations per year (mean difference: 0.79; 95% CI: 0.22-1.36) [11]. 26.6% individuals with COPD reported either night-time and/or daytime gastro-esophageal reflux disease. Patients with GERD had significantly more chronic bronchitis, more breathlessness, and more of them had a history of respiratory infections than individuals with COPD but without gastroesophageal reflux disease [12]. Higher prevalence of GERD symptom, decreased lower and upper esophageal sphincter pressure, increased abnormal distal and proximal reflux, especially non-acid reflux, were found in idiopathic pulmonary fibrosis patients compared with healthy volunteers [13]. GER is reported prevalence ranging from 35 to 81% in patients with cystic fibrosis [14]. Up to 75% of lung transplant patients have demonstrable GERD. Elevated biomarkers, pepsin and bile salts, have been documented in the bronchoalveolar lavage fluid after lung transplantation, suggesting microaspiration [15]. Idiopathic pulmonary fibrosis is associated with increased impedance measures of reflux compared to non-fibrotic disease among pre-lung transplant patients [16]. About 50% of children with recurrent pneumonias and/or clinical asthma were found to have GER, which was reported as an important treatable cause of recurrent pneumonias and/or chronic asthma for those children [17]. When associated with GER, organizing pneumonia is more severe and results in more frequent relapses [18]. Recently, we found some bronchiectasis is also related to GER [19].

GRE was found to be a common risk factor in more and more chronic and refractory respiratory symptoms and diseases causing morbidity and even mortality, indicating that GRE should be well considered, evaluated and treated in chronic respiratory symptoms and diseases.

2. Definition of GERD and Extraesophageal Reflux

In 2006, GERD was defined as a condition which develops when the reflux of stomach contents causes troublesome symptoms and/or complications. The clinical manifestation of GERD was classified was divided into esophageal and extraesophageal syndromes, with extraesophageal syndromes divided into established and proposed associations [20]. The Montreal definition was most extensively accepted, and it is a milestone for clinical practice especially for extraesophageal reflux. In 2013, GERD definition was updated by consensus of the American College of Gastroenterology as a disease comprising symptoms, end-organ effects and complications related to the reflux of gastric contents into the esophagus, oral cavity, and / or the lung [21]. This definition clearly highlighted the reflux affected extraesophageal organs, such as oral cavity, and / or the lung [21].

Extraesophageal reflux is a common problem encountered and called by otolaryngologists as laryngopharyngeal reflux (LPR), LPR is defined as the association of laryngeal symptoms with laryngeal inflammation at laryngoscopy [22].

Independently, based on our own practice and research we developed a concept called gastroesophago-laryngotracheal syndrome (GELTS), GELTS was defined as a series of corresponding clinical manifestations of GER affected upper gastrointestinal tract, airway, ENT and oral cavity, featured as laryngopharyngeal centered airway symptoms, usually asthma, cough and laryngotracheal spasm as its prominent manifestations. In the pathway of GELTS, the gastroesophageal junction act as the generator, the pharynx the reactor, the nose-oral cavity the effector, the larynx and respiratory tract the asthmatic producer, and accordingly GELTS is divided into four phases: gastroesophageal phase, pharyngeal phase, naso-oral phase and laryngo-airway phase [23, 24].

3. Extraesophageal Reflux Effect and Clinical Manifestation

The reflux of gastric or gastroduodenal contents may break through a weakened or damaged lower esophageal sphincter (LES) more easily, dysfunction of the esophageal body may delay esophageal clearance, and hypotonia of the upper esophageal sphincter (UES) may facilitate proximal reflux and transpharyngeal spray into the mouth or airway, which may result in microaspiration and may induce esophageal and/or extraesophageal symptoms [25] through immunological (inflammatory) [26, 27] and/or neural (reflex) [28] pathways.

The esophageal mucosa with its intrinsic anti-reflux defenses can temporarily bear insults of reflux without anatomical modifications of the epithelium, whereas the respiratory mucosa is not resistant to acid injury even in the context of a limited period of exposure. As such, all types of reflux (acid, non-acid, liquid, mixed and air) detected by impedance changes probably should be considered in the diagnosis of LPR. The retrograde flow of the stomach contents up to the throat is associated with many otolaryngological and airway disorders, such as reflux laryngitis, cervical dysphagia, globus pharyngeus, chronic cough, laryngeal or tracheal stenosis, laryngeal carcinoma and asthma. [29-32].

The extraesophageal reflux causes instant irritation first directly onto the upper airway, including a rather wide naso-pharynx cavity with nasal cannels, auditory tube, frontal, maxillary, and sphenoidal sinuses, naso-lacrimal duct, etc., causing sneeze, running or stuff nose, post-nasal drip, tearing, tingling, even hearing disturbance, like symptoms in allergic rhinitis; at the same time or then, the invading reflux micro-particles go into the larynx, trachea, bronchus, and beyond leading to sour throat, especially choking, which means the irritation enters the trachea, causing a series crisis to the patients: asthmatic attack, severe breathlessness, neck tightening, even suffocation. As time goes, this irritation process reaches the lower airways and pulmonary parenchyma causing pulmonary fibrosis and many related lesions [23, 25, 33, 34].

The effect of GER on the concomitant airway symptom in individual is complicated and not easy to identify, GER could be the cause of the airway symptom, or one of the exacerbation factor for the concomitant airway symptom, or only coexistent but not related at all. Based on the anti-reflux outcome of literature and our practice on GER related asthma, we estimated that GER may act as the cause of asthma in 15-25% of the treated cases, the exacerbation factor in 60-70% cases and no related in 10-20% cases [35].

4. Diagnose of Extraesophageal Reflux

The extraesophageal symptom has proven to be highly heterogeneous and the diagnose is very challenging, which often leads to multiple specialty consultations, procedures, pharmaceuticals and diagnostic tests [36, 37]. Traditionally, respiratory and ENT physician are first visited by the patients with extraesophageal symptom, however, the respiratory and ENT physician often had limited tools for diagnose of extraesophageal reflux and limited anti-reflux measures. A small portion of extraesophageal reflux were diagnosed by gastroenterologist, and the treatment was limited to medication therapy [35, 38]. Based on the data published in Chinese literature form 2004-2013, the diagnose of respiratory and ENT diseases constituted 35.28% and 28.61% of the misdiagnose of GERD [39].

The diagnose of extraesophageal reflux should start form the investigation of GER esophageal symptoms, such regurgitation, heartburn and chest pain. The esophageal GER symptoms are present in 59.2% of asthma patients [6], 6-10% of chronic cough patients [40], and 26.6% individuals with COPD [12]. However, up to 10%-62% of GERD related asthma and 75% of GER related cough had unnoticeable GER esophageal symptoms [8], which was called silent reflux [41], so further tests for GER are required.

The extraesophageal symptom is often less specificity, however symptoms such as choking, throat tightness, throat itching, and chronic hoarseness are strongly indicative. The extraesophageal symptom is not season-related in most patients, productive asthma, cough and ENT symptoms often represented in the same individual. The patient has progressive disease without adequate response to respiratory medication. Patent could seldom recall any allergy-inducing factors, but nonspecific factors such as catching a cold or cold air, irritant odors, overeating, irritant or sweet food, lying flat, acid regurgitation or bloating, movement or exertion, and agitated mood are reported to induce the onset of or aggravate the respiratory symptoms. Most of the patients had nocturnal episodes; many patients suffered frequent nocturnal choking, laryngospasm, and/or wheezing during sleep in midnight or early morning. Drinking water, belching or vomiting, adopting a semi-reclining position, or taking an inhaled glucocorticoid or beta-2 agonist helped subdue and reduce the severity of the episodes. Many patients presented with respiratory symptoms that worsened before sleep and were aggravated in the decubitus position, causing difficulty sleeping.

Although current available tests are quite suitable for typical GERD, however these tests have uncertain sensitivity and specificity for the diagnosis of extraesophageal reflux. such as endoscopy, barium study, ambulatory reflux monitoring and high-resolution esophageal manometry are widely used for extraesophageal reflux evaluation, the results should be carefully analyzed.

Reflux symptom index (RSI) and reflux finding score (RFS) were applied during ENT clinical practice. Patients identified by positive results of these tests have a high likelihood of good response to proton pump inhibitor (PPI) treatment [42]. Endoscopy is one of the basic examine for GERD. However, 65% of patients with typical reflux symptoms do not have any esophageal mucosal lesion visible at endoscopy. 30% of patients with reflux symptoms have erosive reflux disease, and 5% have complicated GERD, including Barrett esophagus [43]. Hiatal hernia (HH) also can be detected by endoscopy, the presence HH is more likely to induce GER symptom than patient without HH. 50-94% of the patients with esophagitis were found to have HH, which is significantly higher than that of non-erosive Gastrooesophageal Reflux Disease (NERD) patients (13-59%), and the more sever the esophagitis more HH could be found [44].

Although 24 hour pH-monitoring is one of the current reference-standard methods for GER assessment, it only detects acid reflux. A multichannel intraluminal impedance and pH (MII-pH) monitoring, which detect anterograde or retrograde acid or non-acid bolus and determine the composition, might be more sensitive for GER [45]. Oropharyngeal pH monitoring has been designed for detecting of extraesophageal acid reflux, the test has been found be of highly specificity and can be a helpful reference for anti-reflux therapy [46, 47]. The prolonged wireless pH monitoring is a new technique to monitor esophageal acid exposure, which interfering less with overall daily activities, eating and sleep, and more tolerable and sensitive for acid reflux [48, 49].

High-resolution esophageal manometry is also recommended for fundoplication candidates. high-resolution esophageal manometry is sensitive for LES and UES hypotonic and transit dysfunction of the esophagus. High-resolution esophageal manometry is also a valuable tool for detecting of HH [50]. Barium study is easy to perform and can be well tolerated, it is valuable for primary inspection of esophageal function, obstruction and HH.

The sensitivity and specificity of PPI diagnostic therapy (or so called PPI trial) for typical GERD is as high as 78% and 54% [51]. PPI has also been a diagnostic tool for patients with extraesophageal symptom, and higher dose PPI (twice daily) has been recommended. A good response to a 2-3 month course of PPI treatment may permit a more confident diagnosis of extraesophageal symptom and failure to respond should prompt a more careful re-assessment of the patient [35, 37]. However PPI is much less sensitivity for extraesophageal symptoms than typical GERD symptoms [6, 8], in this term, a negative response to PPI cannot deny the diagnose of extraesophageal reflux [35, 52].

Various biomarkers in different types of biosamples have been studied in the context of extraesophageal reflux; however, they are still not available for routine clinical practice. Inflammatory biomarkers differ in asthmatics based on reflux status. For example, tachykinins are elevated in patients with GERD-related cough and bile acids are elevated in lung transplant patients with

GERD. However, studies like these are often limited by their small size, methods of analysis and case selection. Bronchoalveolar lavage is too invasive to be of use in most patients; exhaled breath condensate samples need further evaluation and standardization and the particles in exhaled air measurements need to be studied further. It is clear that a reliable test to identify GERD-induced respiratory disorders needs to be developed [53]. Recently, pepsin and bile acids were found to be a useful noninvasive marker in the diagnosis of extraesophageal reflux [54-56].

5. Treatment of Extraesophageal Reflux and Outcome

Anti-reflux strategies focus on three main areas: lifestyle interventions, agents to reduce acid or secretion and surgical intervention to reconstruct the esophageal anti-reflux barrier and prevent damage to the esophagus and airway from long-term or repeated exposure to reflux contents.

Lifestyle intervention is an important part of GERD therapy, including weight loss for overweight or have had recent weight gain, head of bed elevation, tobacco and alcohol cessation, avoidance of late-night meals, and cessation of foods that can potentially aggravate reflux.

PPI treatment is commonly recommended for suspected GERD-related asthma, cough and globus, some patients may respond well to PPI therapy. A study over a median of 32 months follow-up, A total of 54% of patients reported improvement of symptom [36]. However, studies to date have shown only limited benefits for the treatment of symptomatic GERD on asthma outcomes and many well-designed studies have failed to demonstrate clear benefit on asthma control [7, 57, 58]. PPIs twice daily sometimes with a prokinetic agent are also recommended for GERD-related chough. It can take more than 50 days for cough to respond to medical GER therapy. In selected cough patients, the responder varies from 56% to 100% in different studies, and in one of the long term study cough improvement in 83% at 6 months, 74% at 2 years and 71% of patients at 5 years [8]. The presence of a pathological acid exposure time or pathological impedance baseline in MII-pH monitoring is associated with a greater probability of PPI response in chronic cough patients [59]. However there was no effect of acid suppression therapy on cough in patients with idiopathic pulmonary fibrosis, and non-acid reflux is increased following the use of acid suppression therapies [60]. Among individuals with COPD exacerbations and coexisting night-time and daytime GER symptom. Approximately 31% of their exacerbations was estimated attributed to lack of regular acid inhibitory treatment [12].

Acid suppression is effective for some individual with extraesophageal symptom, at least 3 months is considered mandatory for adequate course of therapy, maintenance or long term treatment may also required in part of the patients. And the potential reasons for the insufficiency or failure of PPI treatment to elicit a response include non-acid sensitive symptom, inadequate acid suppression , impaired gastric accommodation, delayed gastric emptying, nocturnal gastric acid breakthrough and rapid drug metabolism. In addition, reflux of non-acidic gastric contents (e.g., pepsin, bile acids and pancreatic enzymes), mechanical distention of the esophagus or sensory nerve hyperalgesia may act as a predominant mechanism in eliciting symptoms in the patients that is resistant to PPI treatment. So more effective anti-reflux regimen is required for these patients.

In developed countries, laparoscopic fundoplication (LF) is commonly used for resolving persistent symptoms of heartburn and regurgitation in GERD, especially when it is refractory to PPI treatment [61, 62], and radiofrequency energy application to the gastroesophageal junction is another potentially effective therapy for GRED, even for extraesophageal reflux [63-67]. LF has been recommended by gastrointestinal and endoscopic surgeons for patients with extra-esophageal manifestations (asthma, hoarseness, cough, chest pain, aspiration), especially with evidence of volume regurgitation or any sizable hiatal hernia. LF is safe with fewer complications, especially when performed by skilled surgeons with extensive experience in this procedure [68, 69]. Studies of the outcomes of surgical treatment may be harder to interpret in the tradition of evidence-based medicine as they suffer from a lack of controls and blinding. However, surgical restoration of the anatomical antireflux barrier at the gastroesophageal junction is a more effective method of avoiding any type of GER theoretically and is superior to PPI therapy. A failure of PPI treatment may only mean that acid inhibition for reflux was insufficient to provide a therapeutic effect in some patients and that surgical intervention could be a better choice after careful evaluation [52].

Many uncontrolled studies have been undertaken to investigate the effect of anti-reflux surgery on GER-related asthma outcome. The results of these studies suggest that surgery could improve asthma symptoms and medication use in 80-90% of asthmatics and could also improve pulmonary function in approximately 25%. In these reports, a small proportion of the patients were “cured” of their asthmatic symptoms without any medication [70]. However, there are only a small number of controlled studies. Sontag et al. [71] compared fundoplication to ranitidine and to placebo in asthma patients with GERD. Asthma symptoms and medication requirements improved postoperatively but peak expiratory flow only improved by 10% in one third of the patients. This study was never published as a complete report. A second controlled study with cimetidine noted that drug therapy and surgery for GERD were both associated with an improvement in asthma symptoms and medication requirement at 6 months but not with any statistical significant improvement in pulmonary function compared with placebo [72]. A third study, again assessing ranitidine, showed that 74.9% of patients in the surgery group improved compared with 9.1% of the medical group and 4.2% of the control group [73]. Recently, Sontag et al. [73] compared floppy Nissen to Toupet fundoplication. Symptom scores of cough, asthma, hoarseness and distortion of taste had similar substantial improvements at 3 and 12 months follow-up after surgery. For children, a study by Khoshoo et al. [74] found that PPI/prokinetics or fundoplication in older children with GERD and persistent asthma resulted in a significant reduction in the requirement for asthma medications. Another controlled study by Khoshoo et al. [75] found fundoplication and esomeprazole/metoclopramide to be associated with significantly fewer exacerbations of asthma symptoms in children with moderate persistent asthma and concomitant GERD when contrasted with ranitidine treatment. Recently, a study by Rothenberg et al. [76] examined the laparoscopic fundoplication (LF) outcome of 235 children with severe steroid-dependent asthma and medically refractory GERD. A significant subjective improvement in respiratory symptoms was noted by 215 patients (91%) by the time of the first postoperative visit at 2 weeks. 80% were successfully weaned off their oral steroids within the first 2 postoperative months and 95% reported a decrease in their inhaler use. A symptomatic improvement at follow-up (2 to 72 months postoperatively, with an average of 48 months) was noted by 89% and 99% of those with nocturnal asthma observed a disappearance or significant decrease in their nighttime symptoms. No intraoperative complications or postoperative respiratory tract infections occurred.

LF was also applied on GER related cough. Long tern study by Allen et al. [77], cough improved in 83% (Cured: 52%) at 6 months, 74% (Cured: 43%) at 2 years, and 71% (Cured: 36%) at 5 years after LF. LF is also highly effective in the control of reflux cough in cystic fibrosis, exacerbation events were reduced by 50% post operatively [78]. Some patients with persistent troublesome cough following fundoplication reflux was found to have persistent gaseous reflux on pharyngeal pH monitoring [79]. LF may be efficacious when intensive medical therapy has failed in selected patients who have undergone an extensive objective GERD evaluation [80].

In related studies, GER and recurrent microaspiration have been noted to be common and often severe among patients with advanced lung disease; following lung transplantation, both GERD and aspiration appear to be risk factors for the development of bronchiolitis obliterans syndrome and selected patients may benefit from antireflux surgery [81, 82]. In our opinion, GER should be evaluated and effective anti-reflux measures done before the lung disease getting so advanced to indicate a lung transplantation.

Total (360°) and partial (270° or 180°) wraps of LF are both reliable, effective for anti-reflux. Total wrap is associated with a higher risk of dysphagia, gas bloat, and increased flatulence. We prefer to offer the total wrap mainly to patients who are young, and without significant motility problems who are more acknowledged and tolerated to the side effects. A partial fundoplication with lower incidence of side effects can be applied in patients with advanced age or significant motility problems. New device such as magnetic sphincter augmentation device and LES electrical stimulator are both found to be anti-reflux effective [83, 84], however their outcome for extraesophageal symptoms is still unknown.

6. GERD Department Practice for Extraesophageal Reflux

In 2006, our department for GERD was established by one of the authors of the present study; the author suffered from life-threatening asthma episodes that were completely relieved by LF rather than by asthma treatment regimen [85]. Since then, we recruit, diagnose and treated extraesophageal reflux with anti-reflux medication, radiofrequency energy delivery to the lower esophageal sphincter (Stretta radiofrequency procedure) or laparoscopic fundopliation independently; more than 2000 cases, most of then GER relate asthma, have been documented to date [6, 7].

Our study of LF on extraesophageal symptoms showed an excellent outcome with respect to respiratory symptoms after surgery in 35.9% of cases, a good outcome in 43.8%, fair in 7.8% and poor in 12.5%; accordingly, the mean respiratory symptom score decreased from 6.3 ± 2.65 to 2.33 ± 2.37 at a mean follow-up of 12 months [86]. Our surgical outcome was similar to that reported by other groups [70]. Another study of the Stretta radiofrequency procedure (SRP) for 505 patients with wheezing and chronic cough resulted in a wheezing score reduction from 7.83 to 3.07, a cough score reduction from 6.77 to 2.85, and heartburn score reduction from 5.31 to 1.79 ($P < 0.01$) at a mean follow-up of 12 months [67]. Recently, the five year outcome of the Stretta radiofrequency procedure was reported. The heartburn, regurgitation, chest pain, cough and asthma scores were all significantly decreased compared with the corresponding values before the procedure ($P < 0.001$). After the SRP, 59 (42.8%) patients achieved complete PPI therapy independence and 104 (75.4%) patients were completely or partially satisfied with their GERD symptom control. No prolonged severe complications were observed [64]. Comparing the long term outcomes of the Stretta radiofrequency procedure and LF, we found that both LF and the SRP are capable of controlling symptoms effectively and safely in selected patients; LF gave more improvement in regurgitation, heartburn, chest pain, belching, hiccupping, cough, asthma and PPI elimination, whereas the SRP is less invasive [66, 87, 88]. We also found that the SRP and LF are both effective treatments for GERD-related childhood-to-adult persistent asthmatic patients who had an inadequate response to medical treatment for asthma [65]. Two children who had difficult-to-treat asthma were cured by antireflux interventions [89]; active antireflux treatments can also be beneficial for patients with bronchiectasis and cough syncope, reducing their disabling respiratory symptoms [19, 87].

Conclusion

The pathophysiology of extraesophageal symptoms and GERD, as well as the relationships between them, is much more complex and far from being adequately elucidated. Data from preliminary studies are now available to support the concept that many chronic respiratory diseases, such as asthma and cough, could be induced or exacerbated by GER. However, the causative mechanisms are very difficult to evaluate. We should take into mind that endoscopy, ambulatory reflux monitoring, laryngoscopy, esophageal manometry and PPI trials all have limited utility in the comprehensive evaluation of extraesophageal reflux. Therefore the diagnosis of extraesophageal symptoms is therefore still experimental. High dose with long course of PPI treatment is recommended for extraesophageal symptoms. Preferably done by a skilled, experienced surgeon, LF is found to be somehow practical and more effective for extraesophageal symptoms, and radiofrequency procedure is also a potentially valuable treatment for extraesophageal symptoms.

Conflict of interest: the authors have no conflicts of interest relevant to this manuscript

REFERENCES

[1] El-Serag HB, Sweet S, Winchester CC, Dent J. Update on the epidemiology of gastro-oesophageal reflux disease: a systematic review. *Gut* 2014; *63*(6): 871-80.

[2] Tack J, Becher A, Mulligan C, Johnson DA. Systematic review: the burden of disruptive gastro-oesophageal reflux disease on health-related quality of life. *Aliment Pharmacol Ther* 2012; *35*(11): 1257-66.

[3] Min YW, Lim SW, Lee JH, et al. Prevalence of Extraesophageal Symptoms in Patients With Gastroesophageal Reflux Disease: A Multicenter Questionnaire-based Study in Korea. *J Neurogastroenterol Motil* 2014; *20*(1): 87-93.

[4] Groome M, Cotton JP, Borland M, McLeod S, Johnston DA, Dillon JF. Prevalence of laryngopharyngeal reflux in a population with gastroesophageal reflux. *Laryngoscope* 2007; *117*(8): 1424-8.

[5] Kamani T, Penney S, Mitra I, Pothula V. The prevalence of laryngopharyngeal reflux in the English population. *Eur Arch Otorhinolaryngol* 2012.

[6] El-Serag HB, Havemann BD, Henderson CA. The association between gastro-oesophageal reflux disease and asthma: a systematic review. *Gut* 2007; *56*(12): 1654-64.

[7] Ozcan C, Erkocoglu M, Civelek E, et al. The relationship between gastro-oesophageal reflux disease and asthma during childhood. *Allergol Immunopathol (Madr)* 2014; *42*(2): 109-14.

[8] Chandra KM, Harding SM. Therapy Insight: treatment of gastroesophageal reflux in adults with chronic cough. *Nat Clin Pract Gastroenterol Hepatol* 2007; *4*(11): 604-13.

[9] Bohnhorst I, Jawad S, Lange B, Kjeldsen J, Hansen JM, Kjeldsen AD. Prevalence of chronic rhinosinusitis in a population of patients with gastroesophageal reflux disease. *American journal of rhinology & allergy* 2015; *29*(3): e70-4.

[10] Zelenik K, Matousek P, Formanek M, Urban O, Kominek P. Patients with chronic rhinosinusitis and simultaneous bronchial asthma suffer from significant extraesophageal reflux. *International forum of allergy & rhinology* 2015; *6*(6): 1-6.

[11] Sakae TM, Pizzichini MM, Teixeira PJ, da Silva RM, Trevisol DJ, Pizzichini E. Exacerbations of COPD and symptoms of gastroesophageal reflux: a systematic review and meta-analysis. *J Bras Pneumol* 2013; *39*(3): 259-71.

[12] Ingebrigtsen TS, Marott JL, Vestbo J, Nordestgaard BG, Hallas J, Lange P. Gastro-esophageal reflux disease and exacerbations in chronic obstructive pulmonary disease. *Respirology* 2015; *20*(1): 101-7.

[13] Gao F, Hobson AR, Shang ZM, et al. The prevalence of gastro-esophageal reflux disease and esophageal dysmotility in Chinese patients with idiopathic pulmonary fibrosis. *BMC Gastroenterol* 2015; *15*(1): 26.

[14] Robinson NB, DiMango E. Prevalence of gastroesophageal reflux in cystic fibrosis and implications for lung disease. *Annals of the American Thoracic Society* 2014; *11*(6): 964-8.

[15] Robertson AG, Krishnan A, Ward C, et al. Anti-reflux surgery in lung transplant recipients: outcomes and effects on quality of life. *Eur Respir J* 2012; *39*(3): 691-7.

[16] Gavini S, Finn RT, Lo WK, et al. Idiopathic pulmonary fibrosis is associated with increased impedance measures of reflux compared to non-fibrotic disease among pre-lung transplant patients. *Neurogastroenterol Motil* 2015; *27*(9): 1326-32.

[17] Berquist WE, Rachelefsky GS, Kadden M, et al. Gastroesophageal reflux-associated recurrent pneumonia and chronic asthma in children. *Pediatrics* 1981; *68*(1): 29-35.

[18] Gaillet G, Favelle O, Guilleminault L, et al. Gastroesophageal Reflux Disease Is a Risk Factor for Severity of Organizing Pneumonia. *Respiration* 2015.

[19] Hu ZW, Wang ZG, Zhang Y, et al. Gastroesophageal reflux in Bronchiectasis and the effect of anti-reflux treatment. *BMC Pulm Med* 2013; *13*: 34.

[20] Vakil N, van Zanten SV, Kahrilas P, Dent J, Jones R, Global Consensus G. The Montreal definition and classification of gastroesophageal reflux disease: a global evidence-based consensus. *The American journal of gastroenterology* 2006; *101*(8): 1900-20; quiz 43.

[21] Katz PO, Gerson LB, Vela MF. Guidelines for the diagnosis and management of gastroesophageal reflux disease. *The American journal of gastroenterology* 2013; *108*(3): 308-28; quiz 29.
[22] Koufman JA, Aviv JE, Casiano RR, Shaw GY. Laryngopharyngeal reflux: position statement of the committee on speech, voice, and swallowing disorders of the American Academy of Otolaryngology-Head and Neck Surgery. *Otolaryngol Head Neck Surg* 2002; *127*(1): 32-5.
[23] Wang ZG, Wu JM, Liu JJ, et al. Respiratory distress resulting from gastroesophageal reflux is not asthma, but laryngotracheal irritation, spasm, even suffocation. *Chin Med Sci J* 2009; *24*(2): 130-2.
[24] Wang ZG, Liu JJ, Chen X, et al. Discovery of Gastroesophago-larygotracheal Syndrome (GELTS)—Summing-up on treating 200 GERD Patients with Stretta Radiofrequency. *Clinical Misdiagnosis & Mistherapy* 2007; *20*(5): 1-4+99.
[25] Wang Z, Hu Z, Wu J, et al. Insult of gastroesophageal reflux on airway: clinical significance of pharyngeal nozzle. *Frontiers of medicine* 2015; *9*(1): 117-22.
[26] Sacco O, Silvestri M, Sabatini F, et al. IL-8 and airway neutrophilia in children with gastroesophageal reflux and asthma-like symptoms. *Respir Med* 2006; *100*(2): 307-15.
[27] Zhu GC, Gao X, Wang ZG, et al. Experimental study for the mechanism of gastroesophageal-reflux-associated asthma. *Dis Esophagus* 2014; *27*(4): 318-24.
[28] Rosztoczy A, Makk L, Izbeki F, Roka R, Somfay A, Wittmann T. Asthma and gastroesophageal reflux: clinical evaluation of esophago-bronchial reflex and proximal reflux. *Digestion* 2008; *77*(3-4): 218-24.
[29] Zerbib F, Stoll D. Management of laryngopharyngeal reflux: an unmet medical need. *Neurogastroenterol Motil* 2010; *22*(2): 109-12.
[30] Eryuksel E, Dogan M, Golabi P, Sehitoglu MA, Celikel T. Treatment of laryngopharyngeal reflux improves asthma symptoms in asthmatics. *J Asthma* 2006; *43*(7): 539-42.
[31] Passali D, Caruso G, Passali FM. ENT manifestations of gastroesophageal reflux. *Curr Allergy Asthma Rep* 2008; *8*(3): 240-4.
[32] Delehaye E, Dore MP, Bozzo C, Mameli L, Delitala G, Meloni F. Correlation between nasal mucociliary clearance time and gastroesophageal reflux disease: our experience on 50 patients. *Auris Nasus Larynx* 2009; *36*(2): 157-61.

[33] Wang GR, Zhang H, Wang ZG, Jiang GS, Guo CH. Relationship between dental erosion and respiratory symptoms in patients with gastro-oesophageal reflux disease. *J Dent* 2010; *38*(11): 892-8.

[34] Wang ZG, Ning YC, Wu JM, et al. Airway Presentations due to Reflux Gastroesophageal Airway Reflux and Its Misdiagnosis and Mistherapy. *Clinical Misdiagnosis & Mistherapy* 2011; *24*(3): 1-4.

[35] Hu ZW, Wu JM, Liang WT, Wang ZG. Gastroesophageal reflux disease related asthma: From preliminary studies to clinical practice. World J Respirol 2015; 5(1): 58-64 Available from: URL: http://www.wjgnet.com/2218-6255/full/v5/i1/58.htm.

[36] Francis DO, Rymer JA, Slaughter JC, et al. High economic burden of caring for patients with suspected extraesophageal reflux. *Am J Gastroenterol* 2013; *108*(6): 905-11.

[37] Katz PO, Gerson LB, Vela MF. Guidelines for the Diagnosis and Management of Gastroesophageal Reflux Disease. *Am J Gastroenterol* 2013.

[38] Wang ZG, Ning YC, Wu JM, et al. Airway Presentations due to Reflux: Gastroesophageal Airway Reflux and Its Misdiagnosis and Mistherapy. *Clinical Misdiagnosis & Mistherapy* 2011; *24*(03): 1-4.

[39] Wu QN, Liu L, Y. CB, Fan C, Xu Y, S. Analysis of the related literature about GERD patients who were wrong diagnosed that expressed in domestic journals between 2004-2013. *Chinese Journal of Integrated Traditional and Western Medicine on Digestion* 2014; (06): 300-2+6.

[40] Irwin RS, French CL, Curley FJ, Zawacki JK, Bennett FM. Chronic cough due to gastroesophageal reflux. Clinical, diagnostic, and pathogenetic aspects. *Chest* 1993; *104*(5): 1511-7.

[41] Asano K, Suzuki H. Silent acid reflux and asthma control. *N Engl J Med* 2009; *360*(15): 1551-3.

[42] Habermann W, Schmid C, Neumann K, Devaney T, Hammer HF. Reflux Symptom Index and Reflux Finding Score in Otolaryngologic Practice. *J Voice* 2011.

[43] Savarino E, Zentilin P, Savarino V. NERD: an umbrella term including heterogeneous subpopulations. *Nat Rev Gastroenterol Hepatol* 2013; *10*(6): 371-80.

[44] Hyun JJ, Bak YT. Clinical significance of hiatal hernia. *Gut Liver* 2011; *5*(3): 267-77.

[45] Subramanian CR, Triadafilopoulos G. Refractory gastroesophageal reflux disease. *Gastroenterology report* 2015; *3*(1): 41-53.

[46] Vailati C, Mazzoleni G, Bondi S, Bussi M, Testoni PA, Passaretti S. Oropharyngeal pH monitoring for laryngopharyngeal reflux: is it a reliable test before therapy? *J Voice* 2013; *27*(1): 84-9.

[47] Mazzoleni G, Vailati C, Lisma DG, Testoni PA, Passaretti S. Correlation between oropharyngeal pH-monitoring and esophageal pH-impedance monitoring in patients with suspected GERD-related extra-esophageal symptoms. *Neurogastroenterol Motil* 2014; *26*(11): 1557-64.

[48] Penagini R, Sweis R, Mauro A, Domingues G, Vales A, Sifrim D. Inconsistency in the Diagnosis of Functional Heartburn: Usefulness of Prolonged Wireless pH Monitoring in Patients With Proton Pump Inhibitor Refractory Gastroesophageal Reflux Disease. *J Neurogastroenterol Motil* 2015; *21*(2): 265-72.

[49] Wong WM, Bautista J, Dekel R, et al. Feasibility and tolerability of transnasal/per-oral placement of the wireless pH capsule vs. traditional 24-h oesophageal pH monitoring--a randomized trial. *Aliment Pharmacol Ther* 2005; *21*(2): 155-63.

[50] Kahrilas PJ, Bredenoord AJ, Fox M, et al. The Chicago Classification of esophageal motility disorders, v3.0. *Neurogastroenterol Motil* 2015; *27*(2): 160-74.

[51] Numans ME, Lau J, de Wit NJ, Bonis PA. Short-term treatment with proton pump inhibitors as a test for gastroesophageal reflux disease: A meta-analysis of diagnostic test characteristics. *Gastroenterology* 2004; *126*(4): A319-A.

[52] Wang Z, Hu Z, Wu J, et al. Insult of gastroesophageal reflux on airway: clinical significance of pharyngeal nozzle. *Frontiers of medicine* 2014.

[53] Emilsson OI, Gislason T, Olin AC, Janson C, Olafsson I. Biomarkers for gastroesophageal reflux in respiratory diseases. *Gastroenterol Res Pract* 2013; *2013*: 148086.

[54] Sereg-Bahar M, Jerin A, Jansa R, Stabuc B, Hocevar-Boltezar I. Pepsin and bile acids in saliva in patients with laryngopharyngeal reflux - a prospective comparative study. *Clin Otolaryngol* 2015; *40*(3): 234-9.

[55] Hayat JO, Gabieta-Somnez S, Yazaki E, et al. Pepsin in saliva for the diagnosis of gastro-oesophageal reflux disease. *Gut* 2015; *64*(3): 373-80.

[56] Lee AL, Button BM, Denehy L, et al. Exhaled Breath Condensate Pepsin: Potential Noninvasive Test for Gastroesophageal Reflux in COPD and Bronchiectasis. *Respiratory care* 2015; *60*(2): 244-50.

[57] Holbrook JT, Wise RA, Gold BD, et al. Lansoprazole for children with poorly controlled asthma: a randomized controlled trial. *JAMA* 2012; *307*(4): 373-81.

[58] McCallister JW, Parsons J, Mastronarde JG. The relationship between gastroesophageal reflux and asthma: an update. *Ther Adv Respir Dis* 2010.

[59] Ribolsi M, Savarino E, De Bortoli N, et al. Reflux pattern and role of impedance-pH variables in predicting PPI response in patients with suspected GERD-related chronic cough. *Aliment Pharmacol Ther* 2014; *40*(8): 966-73.

[60] Kilduff CE, Counter MJ, Thomas GA, Harrison NK, Hope-Gill BD. Effect of acid suppression therapy on gastroesophageal reflux and cough in idiopathic pulmonary fibrosis: an intervention study. *Cough* 2014; *10*: 4.

[61] Peters JH. Surgical treatment of gastroesophageal reflux disease. *Gastroenterol Hepatol (N Y)* 2014; *10*(4): 247-8.

[62] Frazzoni M, Piccoli M, Conigliaro R, Frazzoni L, Melotti G. Laparoscopic fundoplication for gastroesophageal reflux disease. *World J Gastroenterol* 2014; *20*(39): 14272-9.

[63] Triadafilopoulos G. Stretta: a valuable endoscopic treatment modality for gastroesophageal reflux disease. *World J Gastroenterol* 2014; *20*(24): 7730-8.

[64] Liang WT, Wang ZG, Wang F, et al. Long-term outcomes of patients with refractory gastroesophageal reflux disease following a minimally invasive endoscopic procedure: a prospective observational study. *BMC Gastroenterol* 2014; *14*(1): 178.

[65] Hu ZW, Wang ZG, Zhang Y, et al. A preliminary investigation of anti-reflux intervention for gastroesophageal reflux related childhood-to-adult persistent asthma. *Ann Surg Innov Res* 2014; *8*: 3.

[66] Liang WT, Wu JN, Wang F, et al. Five-year follow-up of a prospective study comparing laparoscopic Nissen fundoplication with Stretta radiofrequency for gastroesophageal reflux disease. *Minerva Chir* 2014; *69*(4): 217-23.

[67] Gao X, Wang ZG, Wu JM, et al. Radiofrequency treatment on respiratory symptoms due to gastroesophageal reflux disease. *Chin Med J (Engl)* 2011; *124*(7): 1006-9.

[68] Stefanidis D, Hope WW, Kohn GP, et al. Guidelines for surgical treatment of gastroesophageal reflux disease. *Surgical endoscopy* 2010; *24*(11): 2647-69.

[69] Richter JE. Gastroesophageal reflux disease treatment: side effects and complications of fundoplication. *Clin Gastroenterol Hepatol* 2013; *11*(5): 465-71; quiz e39.

[70] Field SK, Gelfand GA, McFadden SD. The effects of antireflux surgery on asthmatics with gastroesophageal reflux. *Chest* 1999; *116*(3): 766-74.

[71] Sontag S J, O'Connell S, Khandelwal S. Antireflux surgery in asthmatics with reflux (GER) improves pulmonary symptoms and function [J]. Gastroenterology, 1990, 98: A128.

[72] Larrain A, Carrasco E, Galleguillos F, Sepulveda R, Pope CE, 2nd. Medical and surgical treatment of nonallergic asthma associated with gastroesophageal reflux. *Chest* 1991; *99*(6): 1330-5.

[73] Sontag SJ, O'Connell S, Khandelwal S, et al. Asthmatics with gastroesophageal reflux: long term results of a randomized trial of medical and surgical antireflux therapies. *Am J Gastroenterol* 2003; *98*(5): 987-99.

[74] Khoshoo V, Le T, Haydel RM, Jr., Landry L, Nelson C. Role of gastroesophageal reflux in older children with persistent asthma. *Chest* 2003; *123*(4): 1008-13.

[75] Khoshoo V, Haydel R, Jr. Effect of antireflux treatment on asthma exacerbations in nonatopic children. *J Pediatr Gastroenterol Nutr* 2007; *44*(3): 331-5.

[76] Rothenberg S, Cowles R. The effects of laparoscopic Nissen fundoplication on patients with severe gastroesophageal reflux disease and steroid-dependent asthma. *J Pediatr Surg* 2012; *47*(6): 1101-4.

[77] Allen CJ, Anvari M. Does laparoscopic fundoplication provide long-term control of gastroesophageal reflux related cough? *Surg Endosc* 2004; *18*(4): 633-7.

[78] Fathi H, Moon T, Donaldson J, Jackson W, Sedman P, Morice AH. Cough in adult cystic fibrosis: diagnosis and response to fundoplication. *Cough* 2009; *5*: 1.

[79] Faruqi S, Sedman P, Jackson W, Molyneux I, Morice AH. Persistent Gaseous Airway Reflux: Cause for Failure of Fundoplication in Reflux Associated Chronic Cough? *Lung* 2012; *190*(1): 63-4.

[80] Irwin RS. Chronic cough due to gastroesophageal reflux disease: ACCP evidence-based clinical practice guidelines. *Chest* 2006; *129*(1 Suppl): 80S-94S.

[81] Sweet MP, Patti MG, Hoopes C, Hays SR, Golden JA. Gastro-oesophageal reflux and aspiration in patients with advanced lung disease. *Thorax* 2009; *64*(2): 167-73.

[82] Robertson AG, Ward C, Pearson JP, Corris PA, Dark JH, Griffin SM. Lung transplantation, gastroesophageal reflux, and fundoplication. *Ann Thorac Surg* 2010; *89*(2): 653-60.

[83] Ganz RA. Long-Term Outcomes of Patients Receiving a Magnetic Sphincter Augmentation Device for Gastroesophageal Reflux. *Clinical gastroenterology and hepatology : the official clinical practice journal of the American Gastroenterological Association* 2015: Epub ahead of print.

[84] Rodriguez L, Rodriguez P, Gomez B, et al. Two-year results of intermittent electrical stimulation of the lower esophageal sphincter treatment of gastroesophageal reflux disease. *Surgery* 2015; *157*(3): 556-67.

[85] Wang ZG. It is gastroesophageal reflux disease, not asthma: a case report. *Chin Med Sci J* 2006; *21*(3): 189-93.

[86] Wang Z, G., Ji F, Wu JM, Lai YG, Gao X, Zhang CC. Effect of laparoscopic fundoplication treatment on gastroesophageal reflux disease -related respiratory symptoms. *Front Med China* 2010; *4*: 254:8.

[87] Hu ZW, Wang ZG, Zhang Y, et al. Gastroesophageal Reflux in Chronic Cough and Cough Syncope and the Effect of Antireflux Treatment: Case Report and Literature Review. *The Annals of otology, rhinology, and laryngology* 2014.

[88] Liang W, Wu J, Hu Z, Wang Z, Zhu G, Zhang C. Laparoscopic Nissen fundoplication is more effective intreating patients with GERD-related chronic cough than Stretta radiofrequency. *Minerva Chir* 2014.

[89] Hu ZW, Wang ZG, Wu JM, Tan ST. Anti-reflux procedure for difficult-to-treat asthmatic children, case report and literature review. *Multidiscip Respir Med* 2012; *7*(1): 28.

In: Gastroesophageal Reflux Disease (GERD) ISBN: 978-1-63484-125-2
Editor: Larry P. Cornett

Chapter 3

EXTRAESOPHAGEAL REFLUX AND SLEEP MICROARCHITECTURE DISTURBANCE AND EXCESSIVE DAYTIME SLEEPINESS

Wilfried Böhning*, MD and Else Briese
Sleep Medicine Centre Karl-Hansen-Klinik
Bad Lippspringe, Germany

ABSTRACT

Gastroesophageal Reflux (GER) has a high prevalence. It should be differentiated between the symptomatic reflux and the so called "silent" Extraesophageal Reflux (EER) with dominant ENT-symptoms. Additionally, it should be noticed that there is a high coincidence with Obstructive Sleep Apnea (OSA).

A pilot study shows that the core symptom of OSA Excessive Daytime Sleepiness (EDS) is also similarly common in EER. The background for this is the sleep microstructure particularly in view of the Cyclic Alternating Pattern (CAP) with the different subtypes. Reflux episodes are not linked to respiratory events.

Reflux events are associated with high arousal activity and simultaneously with increased variability of Heart Frequency (HF) and

* Corresponding author E-mail: w.boehning@medizinisches-zentrum.de.

Pulse-Transit-Time (PTT) – similar to respiratory induced arousals. The usual classification of sleep structure is not useful with regard to the EDS.

With respect to the importance of persistent daytime sleepiness in effective nocturnal ventilated OSA-patients, further appropriate investigations are mandatory.

INTRODUCTION

Gastroesophageal Reflux Disease (GERD) and Obstructive Sleep Apnea Syndrome (OSAS) both have a high prevalence and coincidence **rate** [12, 13, 15, 29]. A causal relationship is discussed in a way that apnea-dependant negative pressures are generated with a strong negative thoraco-abdominal pressure gradient, which favours the regurgitation of stomach content into the esophagus [20]. It was shown that the OSAS-specific therapy with nocturnal ventilation has a positive effect on GERD [10]. The validity of this hypothesis is challenged because a regular relationship between apnea or hypopnea and reflux events could not be shown [14]. On the other hand, however, it is also known that GERD may have a negative effect on OSAS and that a consistent anti-reflux-therapy with proton pump inhibitors (PPI) can cause an improvement in the OSAS-specific symptoms [7].

Repeated reflux events in extraesophageal spaces lead to tissue swelling and thus to a further impairment of the obstruction in the upper respiratory tract. With a laryngoscopy after 8 weeks, posterior commissure edema and hypertrophy was significantly reduced, and objective and subjective sleep parameters were significantly improved [17].

Excessive Daytime Sleepiness (EDS) is a core symptom of OSAS. In a large cross-sectional multicentric epidemiological study with more than 2200 participants, a close relationship between EDS und GERD was also detected [13, 23]. By means of a full polysomnography (PSG), it was shown that in symptomatic GERD a significant higher arousal-index was apparent, however, in patients with a significantly greater Apnea-Hypopnea Index (AHI) the arousal-index was higher in comparison to the severity of patients without reflux symptoms [11]. Using esophageal pH monitoring parallel with PSG there was a similar expression of arousals or changes to sleep-stage "Wake" in symptomatic and asymptomatic patients without adipositas [18]. In this study, the occurrence of reflux episodes increased during the day and at night during stage "wake."

In contrast, Maestri [16] showed that in OSAS-patients with symptomatic reflux, reflux episodes predominantly were found at night, while in Non-OSAS-patients with symptomatic reflux these episodes were mostly detectable at daytime.

The significance of a sleep-microstructure is that it is perhaps more likely to contribute to a clarification of the relationship with regard to the daytime sleepiness. First investigations show that just the cyclic alternating pattern (CAP) has a special importance in GERD [16]. There was a strong association between the CAP and recorded reflux episodes, and the episodes lasted longer when no CAP occurred.

CAP-Electro-Encephalogram (EEG)-activity represents similar sleep instability and sleep disturbance or both. The CAP-sequence is primarily seen as an arousal phenomenon with the idea that both the sleep maintenance and the sleep fragmentation are included [27].

Cyclic Alternating Pattern Definition

- Repetitive EEG-elements with phases A an B
- Phase B corresponds with basic sleep stage rhythm
- Phase A corresponds with the specific salve-like changes of frequency in EEG
- Occurrence only in NON-REM-Sleep
- Differentiation in 3 subtypes

THE DIFFERENT CAP-SUBTYPES A1, A2, A3

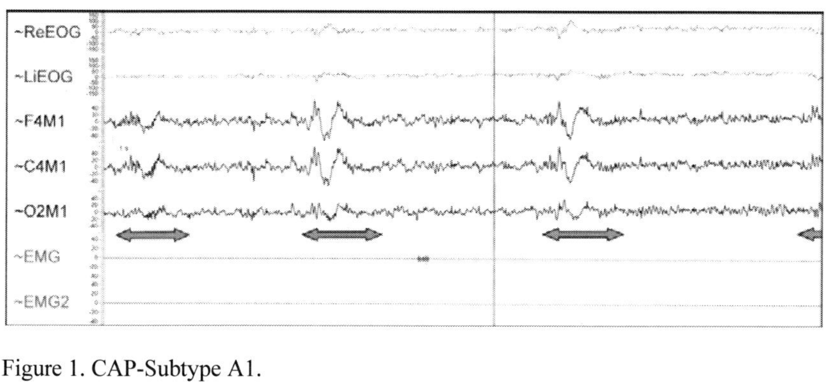

Figure 1. CAP-Subtype A1.

Dominant Delta-activity or K-Complex (synchronized)

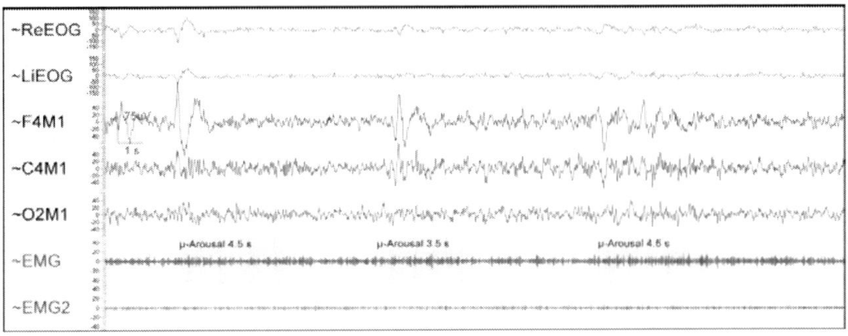

Figure 2. CAP-SubtypeA2.

Beginning with Delta-Waves or K-Complex Merging into Alpha- or Beta-Rhythm (not synchronized).

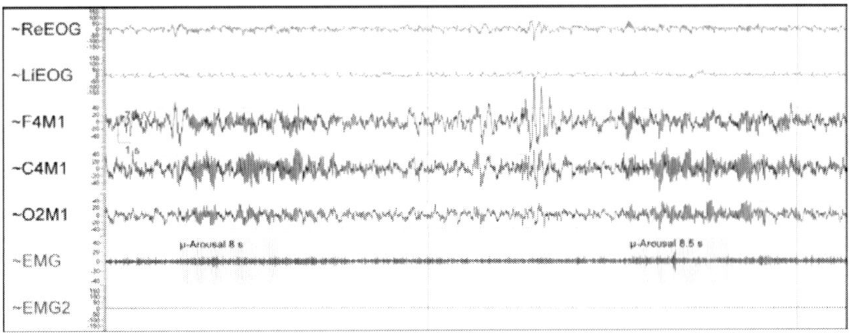

Figure 3. CAP-Subtype A3.

Dominant Alpha- or Beta-Rhythm (not synchronized)

CAP with the two different phases A and B is divided into the 3 subtypes A1, A2 and A3, and their significance for neuro-cognitive functions is very different [26].

The subtype A1 with typical slow wave activity (SWA) as a sign of synchronisation seems to be an expression of cerebral regulation of the effort to maintain sleep. However, if the sleep is increasingly unstable, it comes to desynchronisation with change of the high amplitude SWA to graphic elements of high frequency according to subtypes A2 und A3.

The aim of the study *"EDS in OSAS and Upper Airways Resistance Syndrom (UARS) – Disturbed Sleep Microarchitecture by CAP-Subtypes A2/A3 as a Result of Extraesophageal Reflux*" was to evaluate how frequently an extraesophageal reflux without typical symptoms is detectable in patients with EDS, who were admitted in the sleep laboratory for evaluation and initiation of therapy in OSAS after preceding outpatient cardiorespiratory monitoring and to what extent the sleep microstructure is of importance.

The special technique of reflux monitoring in the assessment of the relationship between OSAS and GERD should be background of this investigation, too.

A reflux demonstrable laryngopharyngeal may be more important with regard to arousals and change from sleep to"Wake" than in the lower esophagus, especially because the intraesophageal placed catheter misses the detection of pharyngeal reflux [26].

Patients with laryngeal reflux very often primarily consult ENT-departments because of the dominant symptoms. As a consequence, these symptoms should be asked for with the specific questionnaire by Belafsky [3].

Table 1. The Belafsky Reflux Symptom Index (RSI)

Finding					
Within the last MONTH, how did the following problems affect you? 0 (none) to 5 (severe)					
1. Hoarseness or a problem with your voice		2	3	4	5
2. Clearing your throat		2	3	4	5
3. Excess throat mucus or postnasal drip		2	3	4	5
4. Difficulty swallowing food, liquids, or pills		2	3	4	5
5. Coughing after you ate or after lying down		2	3	4	5
6. Breathing difficulties or choking episodes		2	3	4	5
7. Troublesome or annoying cough		2	3	4	5
8. Sensations of something sticking in your throat or a lump in your throat		2	3	4	5
9. Heartburn, chest pain, indigestion, or stomach acid coming up		2	3	4	5

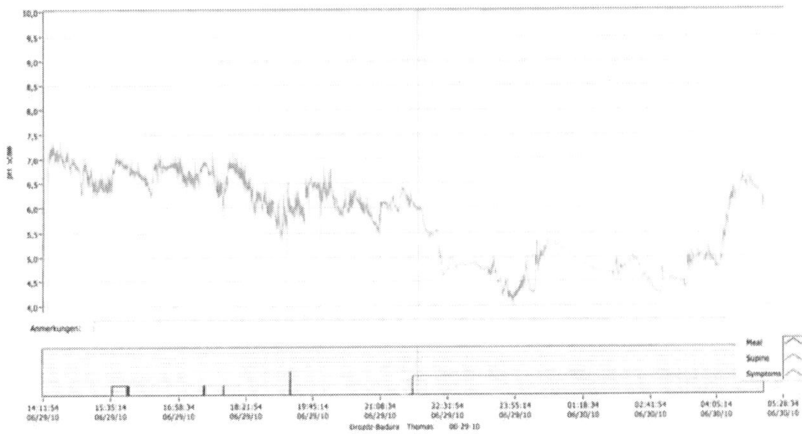

Figure 4. Longterm pH-Metry with Predominantly Nocturnal pH Drop.

The relationship to the validated Reflux Finding Score is well documented [4].

Table 2. The Belafsky Reflux Finding Score RFS)

Finding	Score
Diffuse laryngeal edema	1 = mild
	2 = moderate
	3 = severe
	4 = obstructing
Posterior commissure hypertrophy	1 = mild
	2 = moderate
	3 = severe
	4 = obstructing
Granuloma/granulation	2 = present
	0 = absent
Thick endolaryngeal mucus/other	2 = present
Subglottic edema	2 = present
	0 = absent
Ventricular obliteration	2 = partial
	4 = complete
Erythema/hyperemia	2 = arytenoids only
	4 = diffuse
Finding	Score
Vocal cord edema	1 = mild
	2 = modera
	3 = severe
	4 = polypoid

Patients

11 consecutive patients with EDS (ESS >10, m=10, f=1) mean age 46 years (23-74), BMI 29 kg/m² (25-39) admitted in the sleep laboratory for evaluation of sleep breathing associated disorder (SBAD) and therapy setting.

The study was conducted in June/July 2010.

Exclusion Criteria

Fully vigilance despite pathological polygraphy and complaints of EDS
Symptomatic GERD
Current or within the last 4 weeks PPI-medication regardless of the dose
Limited cooperation or refusal to pH-probe
Intolerance of the pharyngeal pH-probe

Methods

Pupillographic Sleepiness Test (PST, AMTech GmbH, Germany)

Vigilancetest Quatember-Maly, 30-minutes-version (WTS, Schuhfried, Germany)

Belafsky Reflux Symptom Index (RSI)

Full PSG with manual analysis, AASM-criteria (Alice-5-System, Heinen and Löwenstein, Germany)

Simultaneous and time-synchronic epipharyngeal pH Probe (Laryngopharyngeal Reflux, LPR, ResTech DXpH, USA):

Pathologic reflux episode: pH <6,5, % time below threshold >33, drop in pharyngeal pH < 4, 2 times or more [2].

The probe was placed between 12 and 13 pm and pulled usually between 9 and 10 am the following day.

PH measurement was made simultaneously online with PSG.

In addition, continuous pH measurements were done for 20 to 24 hours on an external recorder.

LPR is extremely minimal-invasive and measures the pH in either liquid or aerosolized droplets in the pharynx with known resistance to dehydration but without necessary fluid contact to tissue [2, 9, 24].

Measurement of HF- and PTT-variability, pathologic deviation > 10% compared to before and after the event (both respiratory and pH change induced).

The physiological basis of PTT-changes reflects the variation of the sympathetic tone in response to arousals, and thus is inversely proportional to the blood pressure [8].

RESULTS

The LPR probe was well tolerated by all patients in this minimal-invasive technique. There were no complaints about cough or gag reflex directly related to the advanced placement of the probe into the oropharynx. All pH measurements were evaluated fully.

In all patients, the long-term pH measurements were pathological. Based on the parameters, above we found pronounced acid measurements in 8 patients. In 3 patients, we found predominantly alkaline pH values. In all patients, there was a high arousal index, while these occurred predominantly in form of enteroceptive CAP arousals, the respiratory arousals were significantly lower . Three patients showed only small differences between respiratory and enteroceptive arousals.

Only in one patient with very severe OSAS dominated respiratory arousals, there was a strong relation to often and longlasting apneas.

The further differentiation of the CAP resulted in 3 patients with the vast majority of subtype A3, and in only 1 patient with predominantly subtype A1. The other cases were dominated by subtype A2.

The standard sleep parameters (Wake, N1, N2, N3, REM and arousals) show no abnormalities, the frequently observed alpha-/delta-phenomenon is not scored. The consideration of the CAP arousals with the 3 subtypes show the dominance in sleep phases with little apnea. Only in 1 patient with very severe OSAS, this can not be assessed because of the very high Apnea/Hypopnea-Index (AHI) together with long apneic episodes.

The HF- and PTT-variability were detectable in the same expression in apnea induced arousals as in pH dependant CAP arousals.

Table 3. Respiratory and pH- Events with Arousal Differentiation

			SaO_2 / Arousal						pH	
Name, Age Gender: m/f	RDI total	RDI supine	mini	total	Arousal respirat	Arousal motor.	Arousal enteroceptiv	PH Events	mini	m
M.P., 39, m	17	52	84	28	9	7	12	385	2.8	7.4
T.D-B.,39, m	9	17	87	20	5	2	14	88	4.0	7.3
R.H., 51, m	24	26	84	26	7	10	6	80	4.3	6.6
O.H., 42, m	16	52/REM	81	29	6	11	12	134	2.9	7.7
R.E., 57, m	17	38	93	41	10	7	24	47	3.8	6.6
I.B., 54, f	5	29	90	80	2	5	73	221	2.6	6.5
F.F., 39, m	33	71	75	35	13	12	9	28	6.3 max.8.1	7.2
U.H., 47, m	15	35	91	32	11	6	15	36	3.8 max.8.6	6.7
C.O., 23, m	17	23	90	62	13	10	40	59	6.2 max.8.1	7.1
S.P., 38, m	10	18	88	36	6	5	25	8	7.0 max.8.3	7.8
W.Sch., 74, m	43	57	68	62	40	14	8	7	4.1	7.3

Abbreviations: RDI, Respiratory Disturbance Index; SaO2, arterial Oxygen Saturation

Table 4. Sleep Parameters and HF-/ PTT-Variability

Name, Age, Gender	SPT/TiB SE (%)	SL (min)	%REM	%N3	REM-Latency (min)	HF-/PTT-Variability (Δ > 10%) Subtype A
P.M., 39, m	92	5	13	6	74	+ 3
D.-B., T., 39, m	75	10	18	28	144	- 3
H.R., 51, m	95	10	15	17	140	+ 2
H.O., 42, m	85	35	22	22	61	+ 2
E.R., 57, m	84	10	15	20	77	- 2
B.J., 54, f	72	26	10	21	209	- 3
F.F., 39, m	93	9	24	26	132	- 2
H.H., 47, m	88	13	23	22	47	+ 2-3
O.C., 23, m	84	10	16	18	58	+ 2
P.S., 38, m	86	26	27	23	64	+ 2
Sch.W., 74, m	90	14	7	3	189	- 1(-2)

Abbreviations: HF, Heart Frequency; PTT, Pulse Transit Time; SPT, Sleep Period Time; TIB, Time In Bed; SL, Sleep Latency SE, Sleep Efficiency; N3, Slow Wave Sleep.

Discussion

OSAS and GERD are clearly very often coexisting diseases [14]. This was shown by parallel investigations of PSG and long-term pH measurement. Both diseases and therefore their specific treatment – nocturnal ventilation in OSAS respective PPI-medication with nocturnal body position correction i.e., increase the head end by 15 cm in GERD – can influence one another. Effective nCPAP-therapy (nasalContinousPositiveAirwayPressure) in OSAS leads to an improvement of reflux symptoms [7, 14]. On the other hand, an effective PPI-medication in addition to the nocturnal position correction can reduce the severity of OSAS [21]. The background for the coexistence of these diseases is still not established.

EDS is a core symptom of OSAS and essentially the result of high arousal activity and following sleep fragmentation.

Previous studies have not differentiated between symptomatic and asymptomatic reflux, especially not with regard to the arousal activity [18]. Meanwhile, two variants in reflux are distinguished. First, the acid reflux from the stomach into the esophagus with the typical side effects such as heartburn is mainly associated with an erosive esophagitis and second, the more dangerous "silent" reflux with the documented deleterious effects of acid gases above the upper esophageal sphincter (UES) without typical reflux symptoms is mainly associated with a non-erosive esophagitis [22]. In contrast to the "typical" reflux the "silent" reflux symptoms occur in the throat and upper airways and, nearly as a rule because of imperceptibility, they are not recognized. There are more often complaints of atypical symptoms such as chronic cough, hoarseness, forced hawking, globus sensation or dysphagia [3, 19].

Our studied patients were only slightly overweight, except one patient with significant obesity. Several former studies always assumed a connection of the two diseases OSAS and GERD as a consequence of obesity, this view is certainly eliminated by our study.

The present study confirmed an unexpected high prevalence of GERD in proven OSAS with complained and documented daytime sleepiness. Our consideration pointed in the direction that in some patients with persistent reduction of daytime alertness though effective nocturnal ventilated with CPAP-therapy causes other than previously described could be attributed.

The association between GERD and extraesophageal symptoms is poorly understood and in the past difficult to investigate.

With the new technique of LPR we could show that in 8 of the consecutive 11 patients studied being clinically asymptomatic regarding GERD a pathological acid reflux was measurable in the oropharyngeal area. In 3 of the 11 patients alkaline values were present. The known causes for alkaline pH-values such as inflammation in the upper airways, recurrent otitis, chronic sinu-rhinitis, poor oral hygiene and nutrition were excluded.

The possibility of a duodenic-gastroesophageal reflux with certainly clinically more serious problems and with the possibility of bilirubin-influence on pH values could not be investigated in this study.

In addition, it was also shown that, while a larger portion of the patients had a typical course of the pH values during the day, this was still significantly more distinct parallel to the PSG monitoring during the night. In 2 patients, a reflux could only be detected during the night.

In accordance with previous studies, we demonstrated that reflux episodes occurred rarely in close connection to respiratory events either hypopneas or apneas [18]. Accordingly, Suzuki was able to show that LPR and GERD increases in a light to a moderate OSAS and were less detectable in severe OSAS [25].

Of particular importance, however, appears the type of arousals associated with reflux episodes. When considering only the ASDA criteria (ASDA-

Report, EEG-Arousals: Scoring rules and examples, Sleep 1992, 15:173-184) the described graphic EEG elements would not be evaluated.

Maestri for the first time mentioned a significant association between CAP and reflux episodes [16]. A differentiation of the CAP in the 3 subtypes was not made by him yet. He further indicates that reflux episodes in a high percentage (>90%) of time were not committed to respiratory events.

CAP reflect periodic EEG activities during Non-REM sleep and are characterized by repeated spontaneous events (Phase A) different from the background rhythm of each Non-REM sleep stage (Phase B). This change between the two phases is interpreted as an expression of the arousal-instability/stability [26].

The experimental studies of Ferri were able to demonstrate the different properties of the different subtypes of the CAP [5, 6]. Subtype A1 is clearly associated with a better cognitive function, while subtypes A2 and A3 are associated with impaired neuro-cognitive functions such as verbal fluency, working memory and both delayed recall and recognition of words [1]. The subtypes A2 und A3 are generated in parietal-occipital areas and also coincide with arousals in healthy humans while subtype A1 is generated frontally [5, 6]. Studies on expression of these subtypes and association with EDS are not known. It is noteworthy, however, that in our 11 patients in only 1 case the subtype A1 was present in lower overall expression of CAP activity compared to the others.

Since the CAP events correlated in the same degree as apnea-related arousals with HF- and PTT-variability, perhaps they can equally be regarded as a cause of EDS. The dominance of the CAP events in terms of time with reflux events thus can indicate that when there is persistent EDS despite effective nCPAP-therapy, a reflux disease without any complaints of typical reflux symptoms may be the underlying cause. In our study, we definitely had only clinically asymptomatic patients.

The further clinical coarse of these 11 patients could not be pursued in this pilot study. The significance of the described CAP activity cannot be assessed at this stage of research definitely. In controlled studies with more patients, therefore, will be a follow-up and, where appropriate, the additional benefit of an effective reflux therapy to examine.

The neuropsychologic test batteries of different investigators have repeatedly shown a reverse correlation of the test results to the subtypes A1 and A2, A3 respectively [5, 6]. There are no specific findings regarding the relationship of subtypes A2 and A3 to the different components of attention.

With respect to the importance of daytime sleepiness appropriate investigations are mandatory.

CONCLUSION

Our results show that a "silent" reflux is very common in OSAS. Reflux episodes are not linked to respiratory events. Reflux events are associated with high arousal activity and simultaneously with increased variability of HF and PTT – similar to respiratory induced arousals - with a particular expression of CAP events and especially the subtypes A2 and A3. In addition to the apnea related arousals, the proof of CAP arousals can contribute to daytime sleepiness, which was the ultimate inclusion criterion for this study. The usual classification of sleep structure is not helpful with regard to the EDS.

In larger studies, it should be examined whether this constellation of the described findings directly correlates to reflux events. Accordingly, in addition to CPAP-therapy, an aggressive PPI-medication, should be integrated with the treatment of clinically significant daytime sleepiness.

Conflict of Interest

No potential conflicts of interest

REFERENCES

[1] Aricò D., Drago V., Foster P. S., Heilman K. M. , Williamson J., Ferri R., Effects of NREM sleep instability on cognitive processing. *Sleep Medicine* 2010; 11: 791-798.

[2] Ayazi S., Lipham J. C., Hagen J. A., Tang A. L., Zehetner J., Leers J. M., Oezcelik A., Abate E., Banki F., DeMeester S. R., DeMeester T. R., A new technique for measurement of pharyngeal pH: normal values and discriminating pH threshold. *J Gastrointest. Surg.* 2009; 13(8); 1422-9.

[3] Belafsky P. C., Postma G. N., Koufman J. A., Validity and Reliability of the Reflux Symptom Index (RSI). *Journal of Voice* 2002; 16: 274-277.

[4] Belafsky P. C., Postma G. N., Koufman J. A., The Validity and Reliability of the Reflux Finding Score (RFS). *The Laryngoscope* 2001; 111: 1313-1317.

[5] Ferri R., Huber R., Aricò D., Drago V., Rundo F., Ghilardi M. F., Massimini M., Tononi G., The slow-wave components of the cyclic alternatine pattern (CAP) have a role in sleep-related learning processes. *Neuroscience Letters* 2008; 432: 228-231.

[6] Ferri R, Drago V., Aricò D., Bruni O., Remington R. W., Stamatikis K., Punjabi N. M., The effects of experimental sleep fragmentation on cognitive processing. *Sleep Medicine* 2010; 11:378-385.

[7] Friedmann M., Gurpinar B., Lin Hsin-Ching, Schalch P., Joseph N. J., Impact of treatment of gastroesophageal reflux on obstructive sleep apnea/hypopnea syndrome. *Annals of Otology, Rhinology & Laryngology* 2007; 116(11): 805-811.

[8] Geddes L. A., Voelz M. H., Babbs C. F., Bourland J. D., Tacker W. A., Pulse Transit Time as an Indicator of Arterial Blood Pressure. *Psychophysiology* 1981; 18: 71-74.

[9] Golub J. S., Johns III M. M., Lim J. H., DelGaudio J. M., Klein A. M., Comparison of an oropharyngeal pH probe and a standard dual pH probe for diagnosis of laryngopharyngeal reflux. *Annals of Otology, Rhinology & Laryngology* 2009; 118(1): 1-5.

[10] Green BT, Broughton WA, O`Connor JB: Marked improvement in nocturnal gastroesophageal reflux in a large cohort of patients with obstructive sleep apnea treated with continuous positive airway pressure. *Arch. Intern. Med.* 2003; 163: 41-5.

[11] Guda N, Partington S, Vakil N: Symptomatic gastro-oesophageal reflux, arousals and sleep quality in patients undergoing polysomnography for possible obstructive sleep apnoea. *Aliment. Pharmocol. Ther.* 2004; 20:1153-9.

[12] Ing AJ, Ngu MC, Breslin AB: Obstructive sleep apnea and gastroesophageal reflux. *Am. J. Med.* 2000; 108: 120S-5S.

[13] Janson C. et al. Daytime sleepiness, snoring and gastro-oesophageal reflux amongst young adults in three European countries. *Journal of Internal Medicine* 1995; 237: 227-285.

[14] Kerr P, Shoenut P, Millar T, Buckle P, Kryger MH: Nasal CPAP reduces gastroesophageal reflux in obstructive sleep apnoea syndrome. *Chest* 1992; 101: 1539-44.

[15] Lock lll GR, Tally NJ, Fett SL, Zinsmeister AR, Melton III LJ: Prevalence and clinical spectrum of gastroesophageal reflux: a

population-based study in Olmsted County, Minnesota. *Gastroenterology* 1997; 112: 1448-56.

[16] Maestri M, Bonanni E, Quaranta V, Fabbrini M, Di Coscio E, Parisi M, Rossi M, Parrino L, Terzano MG, Murri L: Sleep microstructure in patients with gastroesophageal reflux and OSAS. *Sleep* 2010, Vol. 33: A297, Abstract Suppl.

[17] Orr WC, JT Robert, JR Houck, CL Giddens, MM Tawk: The effect of acid suppression on upper airway anatomy and obstructive in patients with sleep apnea and gastroesophageal reflux disease. *Journal of Clinical Sleep Medicine* 2009; 5(4): 330-334.

[18] Penzel T, Becker HF, Brandenburg T, Labunski T, Pankow W, Peter JH: Arousal in patients with gastro-oesophageal reflux and sleep apnoea. *Eur. Respir. J.* 1999; 14: 1266-1270.

[19] Richter J. E., Extraesophagealpresentation of gastroesophageal reflux disease. *Semin. Gastrointest.* Dis. 1997; 8: 75-89.

[20] Samelson C. F., Gastro-oesophageal reflux and obstructive sleep apnoea. *Sleep* 1989; 12: 475-6.

[21] Shaheen N. J., Madanick R. D., Alattar M., Morgan D. R., Davis P. H., Galanko J. A., Spacek M. B., Vaughn B. V., Gastroesophageal reflux disease as an etiology of sleep disturbance in subjects with insomnia and minimal reflux symptoms: a pilot study of prevalence and response to therapy. *Dig. Dis. Sci.* 2008; 53: 1493-1499.

[22] Sifrim D., Castell D., Dent J. et al., Gastro-esophageal reflux monitoring: review and consensus report on detection and definitions of acid, non-acid and gas reflux. *Gut* 2004; 53: 1024-1031.

[23] Steward D. L., Pantoprazole for sleepiness associated with acid reflux and obstructive sleep disordered breathing. *The Laryngoscope* 2004; 114: 1525-1528.

[24] Sun G., et al., A new pH catheter for laryngopharyngeal reflux: normal values. *The Laryngoscope* 2009; 119(8): 1639-43.

[25] Suzuki M., Arousals in obstructive sleep apnea patients with laryngopharyngeal and gastro-esophageal reflux. *Sleep* 2010; Vol 33, A179, Abstract Suppl.

[26] Terzano M. G., Parrino L., Sherieri A., Chervin R., Chokroverty S., Guilleminault C., Hirshkowitz M., Mahowald M., Moldofsky H., Rosa A., Thomas R., Walters A., Atlas, rules and recording techniques for the scoring of cyclic alternating pattern (CAP) in human sleep. *Sleep Med.* 2001; 2: 537-553.

[27] Terzano M. G., Mancia D., Salati M. R., Costani G., Dicembrino A., Parrino L., The cyclic alternating pattern as a physiologic component of natural NREM sleep. *Sleep* 1985; 8(2): 137-145.

[28] Wiener G. J., Tsukashima R., Kelly C., Wolf E., Schmeltzer M., Bankert C., Fisk L., Oropharyngeal pH monitoring for the detection of liquid and aerosolized supraesophageal gastric reflux. *J. Voice* 2009; 23(4): 498-504.

[29] Zanation A. M., Senior B. A., The relationship between extraesophageal reflux (EER) and obstructive sleep apnea (OSA). *Sleep Med. Rev.* 2005; 9: 453-8.

In: Gastroesophageal Reflux Disease (GERD) ISBN: 978-1-63484-125-2
Editor: Larry P. Cornett

Chapter 4

OSTEOPATHIC MANIPULATIVE THERAPY IN GASTROESOPHAGEAL REFLUX DISEASE

Leonardo Rios Diniz, PT, DO MRO Br, MSc *
and Wagner Rodrigues Martins, PT, DO MRO Br, PhD
Brazilian Institue of Osteopaathic,
University of Brasília, Brasília, DF, Brazil

ABSTRACT

Gastroesophageal reflux disease (GERD) is a chronic condition that affects a growing number of subjects, and is one of the most prevalent diseases in clinical practice.In the US, it has been estimated that GERD has the highest annual direct costs of all gastrointestinal diseases, at $9.3 billion.

Heartburn is the most predominant esophageal symptom of GERD, while bronchospasm and chronic cough are the most common extraesophageal symptoms.Gastroesophageal reflux disease compromises patient quality of life by requiring modification of the patients' eating habits.The resulting changes in sleep patterns, as well as other various recurrent or lasting long-term symptoms, may limit daily activities.

The digestive system presents a complex anatomic and physiologic relationship, starting at the cranial base with the attachments of the esophagus via pharyngeal tubercle, down to the hyoid bone, the sixth

* Corresponding Author address: Email: lrdiniz@gmail.com.

cervical vertebra (C6), the diaphragm and the lesser omentum; also the liver, spleen, kidney and the greater omentum for the stomach.

The esophagogastric junction (EGJ) is a complex valvular structure that prevents reflux, is composed of the intrinsic lower esophageal sphincter (LES), is situated within the diaphragmatic hiatus, and is surrounded by the crural diaphragm (CD), which provides additional sphincteric compression [7]. It is the main barrier against gastroesophageal reflux, and its function has been attributed to intrinsic LES pressure, extrinsic compression of the LES by the CD, the intraabdominal location of the LES, integrity of the phrenoesophageal ligament, and maintenance of the acute angle between the esophagus and stomach, promoting a "flap valve" function.

Vagal preganglionic efferents innervate the LES smooth muscle, both excitatory and inhibitory innervation. Sympathetic efferents from the spinal segments T6 through T10 are likely primarily nociceptive and potential modulators of LES relaxation induced by the vagus nerve. Thus, the vagus nerve is the prime mediator of LES reflexes.

Osteopathic medicine relies on manual contact for diagnosis and treatment, based on the structural and functional integrity of the body and its intrinsic capacity for self-healing. Osteopathic practitioners use a wide variety of manual techniques to improve physiological function and/or support homeostasis that has been altered by somatic dysfunction, i.e., impaired or altered function of related components of the somatic system; skeletal, arthrodial and myofascial structures; and related vascular, lymphatic, and neural elements.

Dysfunctions at the cranial base, lower cervical vertebrae, thoracic inlet, a compromised CD function, and altered distensibility of the hiatal canal, dysfunctions of the diaphragm, liver and stomach could be considered structural factors leading to GERD. Conversely, dysfunctions of the cranial base and the thoracic inlet could affect the vagus nerve, cervical (C3-C4) dysfunctions could affect the phrenic nerve and alter the movement of the diaphragm and EGJ, and thoracic (between T6-T10) dysfunctions could affect the sympathetic innervation of the LES.

Therefore, a detailed assessment of all aspects related to the LES function, directly or not, would provide useful data to draw an appropriate osteopathic manipulative approach, whether addressed to the innervation zones or to the anatomical structures directly related to the LES.

INTRODUCTION

Gastroesophageal reflux disease (GERD) is a chronic condition that affects a growing number of subjects, and it is one of the most prevalent diseases in clinical practice [1]. In the United States it was estimated that 14 to 20% of adults are affected, based on self-reported symptoms [2], and Sandler et al. (2002) showed that it was the gastrointestinal disease with the highest annual direct costs-$9.3 billion [3].

Heartburn is the most predominant esophageal symptom, bronchospasm and chronic cough the most common extraesophageal symptoms [4]. It compromises patients' quality of life, modifying their eating habits and sleep pattern due to its various, recurrent or lasting symptoms that in the long term will limit their daily activities [5]. Furthermore, its multifactorial nature prevents the complete description of the mechanical, chemical, physiopathological and functional factors that predispose to the disease [1, 6].

Anatomy and Physiology

The esophagogastric junction (EGJ) is a complex valvular structure that prevents reflux, composed of the intrinsic lower esophageal sphincter (LES), situated within the diaphragmatic hiatus and surrounded by the crural diaphragm (CD) that provides additional sphincteric compression [7].

It is the main barrier against gastroesophageal reflux, and its function has been attributed to intrinsic LES pressure, extrinsic compression of the LES by the CD, the intra-abdominal location of the LES, integrity of the phrenoesophageal ligament, and maintenance of the acute angle of His promoting a "flap valve" function. The association of its constituent parts and their ability to maintain a high-pressure zone or a closed luminal segment in the region separating the stomach from the esophagus plays a major role in its global function [8, 9].

The LES smooth muscle is innervated by vagal preganglionic efferents, providing both excitatory and inhibitory innervation to the LES. The sympathetic efferents originate in thoracic spinal segments T6-T10 and they may not exert a major direct effect on LES contraction or relaxation. They are likely primarily nociceptive and potentially a modulator of LES relaxation induced by the vagus nerve. Thus, this latter is the prime mediator of LES reflexes [7].

The CD surrounds the esophagus with a loop-shaped muscle, forming an extrinsic sphincter around the esophagus – the crural sling [10]. Brasseur et al. (2007) observed that the lower esophageal sphincter presents two components, one proximal and another distal. They separated and quantified these components and identified two pressure peaks, one upper peak overlapped and displaced rigidly with the crural sling and one lower peak that likely reflects the gastric sling/clasp muscle fibers at the EGJ [11].

Moreover, Shafik et al. (2005) observed that the crural sling seems to effect esophageal occlusion not only by direct compression but also by "kinking" the esophagus [10].

Pandolfino et al. (2007) using high-resolution manometry, suggested that the compromised CD function, indicated by diminished inspiratory augmentation of EGJ pressure, is an independent predictor of GERD. They also believe that the radial dimensions or distensibility of the hiatal canal or the thickness and elasticity of the CD itself may be significant factors in maintaining CD function [12].

The works of Kwiatek (2011, 2012) showed that inspiratory component of EGJ pressure is the pressure signature of the CD, and that the pressures oscillations at the EGJ high-pressure zone is proportional to the force of diaphragmatic contraction, whether voluntary or not. This corroborates with the papers of Pandolfino et al. (2007), Brasseur et al. (2007) and Shafik et al. (2005) about CD function [7, 13].

Physical Examination

The physical examination should comprise the craniocervical junction, mainly the relationship between the temporal and occipital bones, because it is a potential site of Vagus nerve compression as well as the C1 and C2 vertebrae. Assess the cervical spine, C3 to C5, for possible effects on the phrenic nerve, due its action on the diaphragm. In addition, the fascial relation between the cervicothoracic junction and its effect on the Vagus nerve and esophagus.

The thoracic spine should be assessed for dysfunctions affecting the sympathetic efferents of both esophagus and stomach, upper and lower thoracic respectively, vertebrae and ribs. In addition, the thoracolumbar junction for its effects on the diaphragmatic crura.

The examination of the diaphragm comprises the observation of its symmetry, freedom of movement, and the relationship with the ribs (its attachments) and the xiphoid process. In addition, the balanced movement between diaphragm and stomach (gastrophrenic ligament) should be also assessed.

Additional aspects to be considered when assessing the patient are the presence of previous trauma/injury on the mentioned areas, the presence of hiatal hernia, Barret's, megaesophagus and other conditions the might directly or indirectly affect the function of the diaphragm and the esophagus, and thus, the EGJ junction.

Osteopathic Manipulative Medicine

Osteopathic manipulative medicine (OMM) is based on concepts and unique approaches that are capable of producing the necessary actions to enable the self-healing and self-regulating process within the body[15].

While there are several techniques described in books and in a few research articles, we will describe here mostly the techniques described at the scientific literature.

Smilovicz [16] applied high-velocity low-amplitude (HVLA), balanced membranous tension, muscle energy and myofascial release techniques to the occipito-atlanto-axial (OA) joint, occipitomastoid suture, C2 vertebra and nonneutral thoracic mechanics, but with no specific description of what or how the technique was used in each region.

The work of da Silva et al. [17] showed the effect of a modified diaphragm stretching technique, based on the work of Coster and Pollaris [18], leading to an increase of lower esophageal sphincter pressure after the intervention.

Branyon [19] applied condylar decompression to the OA joint to normalize the parasympathetic tone, myofascial and muscle energy techniques around T5-T9 vertebrae to normalize the sympathetic tone and to release patterns of segmental facilitation and its associated somatic dysfunction, and Celiac ganglion release to normalize hypersympathetic outflow to the upper GI tract.

Mirocha and Parker [20] applied muscle energy and HVLA techniques to the thoracic spine as well as soft tissue techniques to treat functional dyspepsia and reported successful management.

Diniz et al. [21] applied techniques of hiatal hernia reduction [22], pillars of the diaphragm normalization [23], sphincter normalization by recoil [22], and balancing of diaphragms [22], reporting successful reduction of the symptoms.

Stone et al. suggested a gentle inferior traction via a subcostal stomach release, stretching its attachments with the diaphragm, spleen and splenic flexure, or variations of the technique to engage the cardia or the left lobe of the liver [24].

Despite of the positive outcomes shown by the authors cited, providing strong evidence to support OMM as an adjuvant treatment of GERD or other gastrointestinal diseases. There is still a lack of randomized controlled trials with a proper sample and a standardized OMT protocol to understand the mechanism and use of osteopathic manipulative treatment in GERD and other gastrointestinal diseases.

As stated by Steele et al. several issues might compromise the efficacy of OMT studies, like subject recruitment and retention and that the use of standardized protocols is subject to variations among the practitioners. In addition, OMT application cannot always be quantified, especially when treating visceral dysfunctions [18].

References

[1] Moraes-Filho JPP, Navarro-Rodrigues T, Barbuti RC, Eisig J, Chinzon D, Bernardo D. Brazilian Consensus Group. Guidelines for the diagnosis and management of gastroesophageal reflux disease: an evidence-based consensus. *Arq. Gastroenterol.* 2010; 47(1): 99-115.

[2] Kahrilas PJ. Gastroesophageal Reflux Disease. *N. Eng. J. Med.* 2008;359:1700-1707.

[3] Sandler RS, Everhart JE, Donowitz M et al. The Burden of Selected Digestive Diseases in the United States. *Gastroenterol.* 2002; 122:1500-1511.

[4] Vakil NB, Halling K, Becher A, Ryden A. Systematic review of patient-reported outcome instruments for gastroesophageal reflux disease symptoms. *Eur. J. Gastroenterol. Hepatol.* 2013; 25(1):2-14.

[5] Komarchuk VV [Evaluation of quality of life of patients with complicated forms of ulcer in combination with reflux disease]. *Klin. Khir.* 2012 Oct; (10): 62-4.

[6] Velanovich V, Vallance ST, Gusz JR, Tapia FV, Harkabus MA. Quality of life scale for gastroesophageal reflux disease. *J. Am. Col. Surg.* 1996; 183: 217-24.

[7] Kwiatek MA, Kahrilas PJ. Physiology of the LES. *Dis. Esophagus* 2011;25: 286-291.

[8] Delattre JF, Avisse C, Marcus C, Flament JB. Functional anatomy of the gastroesophageal junction. *Surg. Clin. North Am.* 2000; 80(1):241-60.

[9] Pandolfino JE, Kwiatek MA, Kahrilas PJ. The Pathophysiologic Basis for Epidemiologic Trends in Gastroesophageal Reflux Disease. *Gastroenterol Clin. N. Am.* 2008;37: 827-843.

[10] Shafik A, Shafik A, El-Sibai O, Shafik I. Physioanatomic study of the diaphragmatic crura: the identification of autonomous "gastroesophageal sphincter." *J. Invest. Surg.* 2005; 18(3): 135-42.

[11] Brasseur JG, Ulerich R, Dai Q, Patel DK, Soliman AMS, Miller LS. Pharmacological dissection of the human gastro-oesophageal segment into three sphincteric components. *J. Physiol.* 2007; 580(Pt.3): 961-75.

[12] Pandolfino JE, Kim H, Ghosh SK, Clarke JO, Zhang Q, Kahrilas PJ. High-resolution manometry of the EGJ: an analysis of crural diaphragm function in GERD. *Am. J. Gastroenterol.* 2007;102(5): 1056-63.

[13] Kwiatek MA, Pandolfino JE, Kahrilas PJ. 3D-high resolution manometry of the esophagogastric junction. *Neurogastroenterol Motil.* 2011;23:e461-e469.

[14] Michelfelder AJ, Lee KC, Bading EM. Integrative medicine and gastrointestinal disease. *Prim. Care* 2010; 37(2): 255-67.

[15] Posadzki P, Ernst E. Osteopathy for musculoskeletal pain patients: a systematic review of randomized controlled trials. *Clin. Rheumatol.* 2011; 30(2):285-91.

[16] Smilowicz A. An Osteopathic Approach to Gastrointestinal Disease: Somatic Clues for Diagnosis and Clinical Challenges Associated With *Helicobacter pylori* Antibiotic Resistance. *JAOA* May 2013; 113(5): 404-16.

[17] da Silva RCV, de Sá CC, Pascual-Vaca ÁO et al. Increase of lower esophageal sphincter pressure after osteopathic intervention on the diaphragm in patients with gastroesophageal reflux. *Dis. Esophagus* 2012;doi: 10.1111/j.1442-2050.2012.01372.x

[18] Coster M, Pollaris A. Osteopatía Visceral, 2nd ed. Paidotribo, Barcelona, 2005.

[19] Branyon B. Healing hands: using osteopathic manipulative treatment to address visceral structures through somatovisceral reflexes, a case study. *AAOJ* 2008;18: 29-31.

[20] Mirocha NJ, Parker JD. Successful treatment of refractory functional dyspepsia with osteopathic manipulative treatment: a case report. *OFP*2012; 4(6):193-196. doi: 10.1016/j.osfp.2012.01.003

[21] Diniz LR, Nesi J, Curi AC, Martins WR. Qualitative Evaluation of Osteopathic Manipulative Therapy in a Patient with Gastroesophageal Reflux Disease: a Brief Report. *JAOA* 2014;114(3): 180-88.

[22] Quef BH. *Técnicas Osteopáticas Viscerais*. Ed. Santos, São Paulo 2008.

[23] Camirand N. *Dysfonctions glandulaires et nerveuses. Diagnostics et traitements ostéopathiques*. Maloine, Paris 2009.

[24] Stone CA. Visceral and Obstetric Osteopathy. Churchill Livingstone Elsevier, London 2007.

[25] Lossing K. Visceral Manipulation. In: Chila AG. *Foundations of Osteopathic Medicine*. 3rd ed./published under the auspices of the American Osteopathic Association. Philadelphia: Lippincott Williams & Wilkins; 2011: 845-849.

[26] Steele KM, Viola J, Burns E, Carreiro JE. Brief Report of a Clinical Trial on the Duration of Middle Ear Effusion in Young Children Using a Standardized Osteopathic Manipulative Medicine Protocol. *J. Am. Osteopath. Assoc*. 2010;110(5): 278-284.

[27] Shafik A, Shafik I, El-Sibai O, Mostafa RM. Does the crural diaphragm share in the contractile activity of the costal diaphragm? The concept of an "autonomous esophageal crus" and its role in esophageal competence. *Med. Sci. Monit.* 2004; 10(8):BR268-72.

[28] Shafik A, El-Sibai O, Shafik I, Shafik A. Electroesophagogram in gastroesophageal reflux disease with a new theory on the pathogenesis of its electric changes. *BMC Surg*. 2004;4:13.

[29] Shafik A, Shafik I, El-Sibai O, Shafik AA. On the pathogenesis of gastroesophageal reflux: the concept of gastroesophageal dyssynergia. *J. Thorac. Cardiovasc. Surg*. 2005; 130(2):401-7.

[30] Grundy D, Al-Chaer ED, Aziz Q et al. Fundamentals of Neurogastroenterology: Basic Science. *Gastroenterol.* 2006;130: 1391-1411.

In: Gastroesophageal Reflux Disease (GERD) ISBN: 978-1-63484-125-2
Editor: Larry P. Cornett

Chapter 5

GASTROESOPHAGEAL REFLUX DISEASE (GERD): UPDATE IN THE SURGICAL APPROACH AND LONG-TERM OUTCOME

Jaime Ruiz-Tovar[1,*], MD, PhD
and Carolina Llavero[2], RN
[1]Department of Surgery. University Hospital Rey Juan Carlos, Madrid, Spain
[2]Department of Surgical Nursery. Sureste Hospital, Madrid, Spain

ABSTRACT

Gastroesophageal reflux disease (GERD) is a very frequent pathology in developed countries. After failure of initial medical treatment, mainly based on Proton Pump Inhibitors (PPI), surgery is indicated. The goal of antireflux operation is to achieve control of the symptoms with minimum risk and without adding any long-term side effects to the patient undergoing the procedure. Laparoscopic approach has become the elective approach for the surgical treatment of GERD in the last decade. Compared with conventional surgery, laparoscopy presents lower complication and mortality rates, and a shorter hospital stay. There is a great controversy about the fundoplication technique of

---

* Correspondence to: Jaime Ruiz-Tovar, MD,PhD, Corazon de Maria, 64, 7º J, 28002-Madrid (Spain), Tlf: (0034)630534808, Email: jruiztovar@gmail.com.

choice. Nissen funcoplication seems to be the better antireflux technique for some authors, presenting the smaller recurrence rate. However, Nissen fundoplication is also associated with higher incidence of dysphagia, that may reach up to 20% of the cases.

Outcome data beyond 10 years describe good-to-excellent outcomes in most patients. The durability of fundoplication has been documented with more than 90% of patients satisfied after 10 years, without recurrence of reflux symptoms or appearance of dysphagia.

In this chapter we will review the actual evidence about all these issues.

INTRODUCTION

Gastroesophageal reflux disease (GERD) is a very frequent pathology in developed countries. Initial treatment of this entity is medical therapy, which consists of both drug therapy proton pump inhibitors (PPIs) and lifestyle modifications. Surgical management is generally reserved for patients with complications of reflux, such as recurrent or refractory esophagitis, Barrett's metaplasia, persistent "reflux symptoms" despite acid suppression, or asthma. Patients who are unable to tolerate medication, noncompliant with medication, or who are medication dependent and unwilling to take lifelong medications are also surgical candidates [1].

Indications for Antireflux Surgery

Indications for surgery in the patient with GERD can be divided into:

1. Gastrointestinal Indications [1]

- Failed optimal medical management
- Noncompliance with medical therapy
- High volume reflux
- Severe esophagitis by endoscopy
- Benign stricture
- Barrett's columnar-lined epithelium (without severe dysplasia or carcinoma)

2. Non Gastrointestinal Indications

About one-half of patients with GERD report upper respiratory symptoms including hoarseness, laryngitis, wheezing, nocturnal asthma, cough, aspiration, or dental erosion. Relief of respiratory symptoms is usually achievable by fundoplication [2, 3].

Although cough may present as one of the most common extraesophageal symptoms of GERD, asthma, chronic bronchitis, laryngitis, idiopathic subglottic stenosis, and even laryngeal cancer have also been implicated [4]. Many of these patients do not have typical features of GERD, such as heartburn [5].

Preoperative Evaluation

There is no consensus for the optimal preoperative investigation for surgical candidates. Upper endoscopy, esophageal manometry, and pH metry are the most useful tests in making surgical decisions.

- Upper endoscopy: Esophageal and gastric endoscopy should be performed to assess the esophageal and gastric mucosa for signs of malignancy prior to proceeding with a surgical antireflux procedure.
- Esophageal manometry: Esophageal manometry studies should be used routinely in preoperative evaluation. Manometry occasionally provides alternative diagnoses, such as scleroderma or achalasia, for which antireflux surgery may be contraindicated. In addition, manometry might lead to a modification of the surgical approach or a change in management, opting many surgeons for performing partial 270º fundoplications in patients with altered esophageal motility rather than a Nissen fundoplication (360º). However, the need to modify the surgical procedure based upon the manometric findings has been questioned by other authors [6].
- 24 hours-PH metry: Actually considered the gold standard for the diagnosis of GERD. Criteria for this diagnosis are pH <4 during more than 4.5% of the time after 24 hours monitoring and a DeMeester punctuation >14.72.

Antireflux Surgical Techniques

Current experience with antireflux surgery suggests that there is no operation of choice for all patients. Factors such as the degree of esophageal shortening, disturbances of esophageal motility, prior operations, and local expertise with laparoscopic techniques influence the choice of operation. It remains unclear which patient characteristics influence postoperative success following fundoplication for GERD [7].

For the patient with normal esophageal length and motility, the operation of choice is probably a laparoscopic Nissen fundoplication. However, studies comparing partial fundoplication (180º-270º) to the 360º Nissen fundoplication have consistently reported less postoperative dysphagia with partial fundoplication, but greater long-term durability with complete fundoplication [8]. A recent study of our group, including 106 patients with long-term follow up and comparing Nissen fundoplication versus Toupet fundoplication (270º posterior fundoplication), showed that 10 years after surgery 10% of the patients remain symptomatic in both groups and 15% in each group continued with PPI treatment. However, 20% of the patients undergoing Nissen fundoplication complained of dysphagia and 4% required reoperation and conversion to a partial fundoplication (Toupet approach). Patients undergoing Toupet technique did not present dysphagia. Given these results, partial fundoplication obatain similar results to Nissen fundoplication and the risk of dysphagia is lower. Therefore, we recommended a partial fundoplication as the technique of choice for the treatment of GERD [9].

Dysphagia after Nissen fundoplication has been attributed to a narrow hiatus, but many groups calibrate the hiatus with a 36F bougie, but recent opinions suggest that the main cause of dysphagia results from a twisting of the gastric fundus around the esophagus. The most common error in constructing the fundoplication is to grasp the anterior portion of the stomach too low on the major curvature and to pull it behind the esophagus [10, 11]. We do not really know the reason of dysphagia in 20% of our NF patients, but it is high enough in order to choose another technique, especially when the long term results of partial fundoplications are excellent.

Laparoscopy versus Laparotomy

A laparoscopic operation performed by an experienced surgeon can offer significant advantages over the open approach, with similar efficacy and safety. Thus, laparoscopic surgery has become the elective approach for the surgical treatment of GERD in the last decade. Compared with the conventional surgery, laparoscopy implies lower complication and mortality rates, and a shorter hospital stay [12].

Long term reflux control has been shown to be equal to open procedure in some studies [13], but other authors still refer worse results after laparoscopic surgery, with more frequency of postoperative reflux symptoms and disabling dysphagia and less patients satisfied with the procedure in the laparoscopic group compared to the conventional approach [14]. A 2005 systematic review concluded that laparoscopic fundoplication was as effective as open fundoplication for relieving heartburn and regurgitation, improving quality of life, and decreasing antisecretory medications. Almost 90% of patients who were followed for five or more years reported improvement in symptoms [15]. Some studies have suggested that the laparoscopic approach has been associated with a relatively high incidence of postoperative dysphagia (8% - 12%) compared with an open approach. Why this might occur is not well understood. It may be attributable at least in part to difficulty determining the looseness of the wrap at laparoscopy. For this reason, many surgeons construct the wrap over a large esophageal Bougie (48 to 60 Fr) [16].

In our experience, better long term results were obtained after laparoscopic surgery than after an open approach, with less symptomatic patients and less patients taking daily PPI after 10 years follow up [17]. Better results after laparoscopic surgery could be somehow explained because of a better exposure of the hiatus and a more comfortable dissection and performance of the fundoplication during the laparoscopic approach, while the open one presents bad access to the upper parts of the abdomen. A common opinion in the past was that it is more difficult to perform the "floppy" fundoplication by a laparoscopic approach, due to its technically difficulty [9], than with the open technique, but actually this afirmation is not supported any more with the increasing experience of the surgeons in laparoscopic techniques [13, 18].

Long-Term Outcome after Antireflux Surgery

Long-term observational studies of laparoscopic fundoplication by experienced operators generally report that 90 to 95% percent of a patients are satisfied with the results of their surgery, similar results to those obtained by open approach [19, 20]. However, consensus has not been achieved on what constitutes treatment success or failure. It seems logical that continued use of anti-acid medications must be considered a treatment failure. Furthermore, some patients who require anti-acid medications after surgery still report high quality of life compared with preoperative status, as many patients on acid suppression medications do not have documental reflux [21]. As previously mentioned, in our experience, 10% of the patients remained with GERD symptoms and up to 15% continued with their anti-acid medication. This represents a 25% failure of the surgery. However, when investigating the satisfaction rate of the patients, over 95% of them were satisfied or very satisfied.

The comparison of surgical options is a complex topic since there is heterogeneity of techniques and technical choices that may impact outcome. As for many technical procedures, the actual tendency is that the best choice for an individual patient may be the procedure in which the surgeon is most skilled.

When comparing Toupet with Nissen fundoplication, similarly to our results, Mardani et al. performed a randomized trial including 137 patients with chronic GERD and esophagitis undergoing either a partial wrap (Toupet posterior procedure) or a total wrap (Nissen procedure). Patients treated with a partial wrap had equivalent rates of control of symptoms of heartburn (80% vs 87%) and acid regurgitation (82% vs 90%) after a mean of 18 years of observation. Both groups had similar rates of long-term side effects such as bloating, flatulence, and dysphagia scores [22].

In a systematic review and meta-analysis of five randomized trials that included 458 patients, patients undergoing a laparoscopic anterior fundoplication (Dor technique) had a similar heartburn score, dilatation rate, proton pump inhibitor (PPI) use, and patient satisfaction score when compared with patients undergoing a laparoscopic Nissen approach. At one-year, however, patients undergoing a Dor technique had significantly less gas bloating (11% vs 18%), flatulence (14% vs 25%) and inability to relieve bloating (34% vs 44%) [23].

When comparing the laparoscopic anterior fundoplication (LAF) (Dor technique: 180° wrap) with the laparoscopic posterior fundoplication (LPF) (Toupet technique: 270° wrap), a meta-analysis of seven randomized trials found that the short-term results for 338 patients treated by a LPF included significantly less esophageal acid exposure time (0.8% vs 3.3%), heartburn (8% vs 21%), and a lower reoperation rate (4% vs 8%) compared with 345 patients undergoing LAF. There were no significant short-term differences for the rate of esophagitis, regurgitation, belching, lower esophageal sphincter pressure, or satisfaction between the two approaches. The long-term outcomes for patients undergoing a LPF included a significantly lower rate of persistent heartburn (14% vs 31%) and a significantly lower reoperation rate (5% vs 10%), but no differences in dysphagia scores, inability to belch, gas bloating, or patient satisfaction [24].

REFERENCES

[1] Zaninotto G, Attwood SE. Surgical management of refractory gastro-oesophageal reflux. *Br. J. Surg.* 2010; 97:139-140.

[2] Downing TE, Sporn TA, Bollinger RR, et al. Pulmonary histopathology in an experimental model of chronic aspiration is independent of acidity. *Exp. Biol. Med.* (Maywood) 2008; 233:1202-1212.

[3] Lazarchik DA, Frazier KB. Dental erosion and acid reflux disease: an overview. *Gen. Dent.* 2009; 57:151-156.

[4] Johanson JF. Epidemiology of esophageal and supraesophageal reflux injuries. *Am. J. Med.* 2000; 108 Suppl 4a:99S-103S.

[5] Smullen JL, Lejeune FE Jr. Otolaryngologic manifestations of gastroesophageal reflux disease. *J. La State Med. Soc.* 1999; 151:115-119.

[6] Fibbe C, Layer P, Keller J, et al. Esophageal motility in reflux disease before and after fundoplication: a prospective, randomized, clinical, and manometric study. *Gastroenterology* 2001; 121:5-14.

[7] Ip S, Tatsioni A, Conant A, et al. Predictors of clinical outcomes following fundoplication for gastroesophageal reflux disease remain insufficiently defined: a systematic review. *Am. J. Gastroenterol.* 2009; 104:752-758.

[8] Ludemann R, Watson DI, Jamieson GG, et al. Five-year follow-up of a randomized clinical trial of laparoscopic total versus anterior 180 degrees fundoplication. *Br. J. Surg.* 2005; 92:240-243.

[9] Ruiz-Tovar J, Diez M, Chames A, et al. Clinical outcome at ten years after laparoscopic fundoplication: Nissen versus Toupet. *Am. Surg.* 2010;12: 1408-1411.

[10] Kelly JJ, Watson DI, Chin KF, Devitt PG, Game PA, Jamieson GG. Laparoscopic Nissen funduplication : Clinical outcomes at 10 years. *J. Am. Coll. Surg.* 2007;205:570-5.

[11] Bowrey DJ, Peters JH.Current state, techniques and results of laparoscopic antireflux surgery. *Semin. Laparosc. Surg.* 1999;6:194-212.

[12] Geibel J, Longo W. Controversies in the treatment of gastriesophageal reflux and acalasia. *World J. Gastroenterol.* 2006;12:3155-3161.

[13] Bammer T, Hinder RA, Alexander K, Klingler PJ. Five-to-eight year outcome of the first laparoscopic Nissen fundoplications. *J. Gastrointest. Surg.* 2001;5:42-48.

[14] Franzen T, Anderberg B, Wiren M, Johansson KE. Long-term outcome is worse after laparoscopic than after conventional Nissen funduplication. *Scand. J. Gastroenterol.* 2005;40:1261-1268.

[15] Ip S, Bonis P, Tatsioni A, et a. Comparative Effectiveness of Management Strategies for Gastroesophageal Reflux Disease. Evidence Report/Technology Assessment No. 1. (Prepared by Tufts-New England Medical Center. Evidence-based Practice Center under Contract No. 290-02-0022.) Rockville, MD: Agency for Healthcare Research and Quality. December 2005. www.effectivehealthcare.ahrq.gov/reports/final.cfm (Accessed on December 18, 2007).

[16] Bais JE, Bartelsman JF, Bonjer HJ, et al. Laparoscopic or conventional Nissen fundoplication for gastro-oesophageal reflux disease: randomised clinical trial. The Netherlands Antireflux Surgery Study Group. *Lancet* 2000; 355:170-174.

[17] Ruiz-Tovar J, Diez M, Chames A, et al. Clinical outcome at years after laparoscopic versus open Nissen fundoplication. J Laparoendosc Adv Surg Tech 2010; 20:21-23.

[18] Mehta S, Boddy A, Rhodes M. Review of outcome after laparoscopic paraesophageal hiatal hernia repair. *Surg. Laparosc. Endosc. Percutan. Tech.* 2006; 16:301-306.

[19] Dassinger MS, Torquati A, Houston HL, et al. Laparoscopic fundoplication: 5-year follow-up. *Am. Surg.* 2004; 70:691-694.

[20] Cowgill SM, Arnaoutakis D, Villadolid D, et al. Results after laparoscopic fundoplication: does age matter? *Am. Surg.* 2006; 72:778-783.

[21] Lord RV, Kaminski A, Oberg S, et al. Absence of gastroesophageal reflux disease in a majority of patients taking acid suppression medications after Nissen fundoplication. *J. Gastrointest. Surg.* 2002; 6:3-9.

[22] Mardani J, Lundell L, Engström C. Total or posterior partial fundoplication in the treatment of GERD: results of a randomized trial after 2 decades of follow-up. *Ann. Surg.* 2011; 253:875-878.

[23] Broeders JA, Roks DJ, Ahmed Ali U, et al. Laparoscopic anterior 180-degree versus nissen fundoplication for gastroesophageal reflux disease: systematic review and meta-analysis of randomized clinical trials. *Ann. Surg.* 2013; 257:850-859.

[24] Broeders JA, Roks DJ, Ahmed Ali U, et al. Laparoscopic anterior versus posterior fundoplication for gastroesophageal reflux disease: systematic review and meta-analysis of randomized clinical trials. *Ann. Surg.* 2011; 254:39-47.

In: Gastroesophageal Reflux Disease (GERD) ISBN: 978-1-63484-125-2
Editor: Larry P. Cornett

Chapter 6

BIBLIOGRAPHY

A practical guide to reflux: causes, consequences, and care LCCN: 2011020173 Main title: A practical guide to reflux: causes, consequences, and care— John W. Birk, editor. Published/ Created: New York: Nova Science Publishers, c2012. Description: viii, 88 p.: ill.; 23 cm. ISBN: 9781613249222 (softcover: alk. paper) 1613249225 (softcover: alk. paper) LC classification: RC815.7 .P73 2012 Related names: Birk, John W. Contents: Gastroesophageal reflux disease: incidence and epidemiology— Deepika Devuni -- Causes and consequences of GERD— Marcy Coash -- Diagnosis of GERD— Maria Johnson -- Treatment of GERD— Priya Rangasamy. Subjects: Gastroesophageal reflux. Gastroesophageal Reflux. Notes: Includes bibliographical references and index. Series: Digestive diseases--research and clinical developments Digestive diseases--research and clinical developments series.

Acid reflux diet & cookbook for dummies LCCN: 2014935507 Personal name: Raymond, Patricia (Gastroenterologist) Main title: Acid reflux diet & cookbook for dummies— by Dr. Patricia Raymond and Michelle Beaver. Published/Produced: Hoboken, NJ: For Dummies, a Wiley brand, [2014] ©2014 Description: xvi, 309 pages, [8] pages of plates: illustrations (some color); 24 cm. ISBN: 9781118839195 (pbk.) 1118839196 (pbk.) LC classification: RC815.7 .R39 2014 Portion of title: Acid reflux diet and cookbook for dummies

Related names: Beaver, Michelle (Health writer) Summary: Put an end to acid reflux-- and take your life back. Raymond and Beaver outline the lifestyle and diet modifications that prevent symptoms from occurring, as well as explanations of the condition and how and why these modifications help. -- Source other than Library of Congress. Contents: Introduction -- Getting started with the acid reflux diet -- Making diet and lifestyle changes -- Symptom-soothing recipes -- Solutions for specific situations -- The part of tens. Subjects: Gastroesophageal reflux. Heartburn. Gastroesophageal reflux--Diet therapy. Heartburn--Diet therapy. Gastroesophageal reflux--Diet therapy--Recipes. Heartburn--Diet therapy--Recipes. Notes: Includes index. Series: --For dummies --For dummies.

Asthma: comorbidities, coexisting conditions, and differential diagnosis LCCN: 2013033500 Uniform title: Asthma (Lockey) Main title: Asthma: comorbidities, coexisting conditions, and differential diagnosis— edited by Richard F. Lockey, MD, Distinguished University Health Professor, Professor of Medicine, Pediatrics & Public Health, Joy McCann Culverhouse Chair of Allergy and immunology, Director, Division of Allergy and Immunology, Department of Internal Medicine, University of South Florida College of Medicine, James A. Haley Veterans' Hospital, Tampa, Florida, Dennis K. Ledford, MD, Professor, Medicine & Pediatrics, Mabel & Ellsworth Simmons Professor of Allergy & Immunology, Division of Allergy and Immunology, Department of Internal Medicine, University of South Florida College of Medicine, James A. Haley Veterans' Hospital, Tampa, Florida. Published/Produced: Oxford; New York: Oxford University Press, [2014] ©2014 Description: xx, 481 pages: illustrations (some color); 27 cm ISBN: 9780199918065 (hbk.: acid-free paper) 9780199918072 (hbk.: acid-free paper) LC classification: RC591 .A78 2014 Related names: Lockey, Richard F., editor of compilation. Ledford, Dennis K., 1950- editor of compilation. World Allergy Organization, issuing body. Contents: Hypersensitivity pneumonitis— David I. Bernstein -- Anti-neutrophil cytoplasmic antibody (ANCA) positive vasculitis— Lanny J. Rosenwasser -- Allergic bronchopulmonary aspergillosis (ABPA)— Paul A. Greenberger -- Immunodeficiency: innate, primary and secondary— John W. Sleasman and Jean M. Brown -- Sleep apnea - comorbid and coexisting - in children and the upper airway— Athanasios Kaditis -- Asthma and obstructive sleep apnea— Larry Ladi and Edward S. Schulman -- COPD and irreversible airflow obstruction— Stephen P. Peters -- Bronchiectasis— Nizar Naji and Paul M OByrne -- Bronchiolitis— Theresa W. Guilbert and Kelly J. Cowan -- Genetic disorders and asthma— Neetu Talreja and Ronald Dahl -- Other pulmonary abnormalities— Robert A. Wise and Emily P. Brigham -- Pneumonia: comorbid and co-existing— Chrysanthi L. Skevaki, Athanassios Tsakris, and Nikolaos G. Papadopoulos -- Cough— Pramod Kelkar, Alan Goldsobel, and Riccardo Polosa -- Occupational asthma comorbid and differential diagnosis— Manon Labrecque, Denyse Gautrin, Ignacio Ansotegui, Roberto Castano, and Gregory Moullec -- Adult cardiac conditions— Paola Rogliani, Andrea Segreti, and Mario Cazzola -- Pediatric cardiac conditions: coexisting and differential diagnosis— Louis I. Bezold -- Pulmonary hypertension— Aaron B. Waxman and Kerri Akaya Smith -- Allergic rhinitis— Robert M. Naclerio and Ruby Pawankar -- Nonallergic rhinopathies and lower airway syndromes— James N. Baraniuk, Michael S. Blaiss, and Debendra Pattanaik -- Infectious comorbidities of asthma in the upper airway— Claus Bachert and Griet Vandeplas -- Nasal polyps: comorbid— Hae-Sim Park, Mario Sanchez-Borges, Marek Kowalski, Seung Youp Shin -- Vocal cord dysfunction and paradoxical vocal fold motion disorder— Roger W. Fox and Mark C. Glaum -- Gastroesophageal reflux— Promila Banerjee and Stephen J. Sontag -- Obesity and asthma— Erick Forno, Louis-Philippe Boulet, and Juan C. Celedón -- Endocrine disorders: comorbid and coexisting— Kyriaki Sideri and Adnan Custovic -- Osteopenia and osteoporosis: comorbidities of asthma— Joshua A. Steinberg and Andrea J. Apter -- Pregnancy comorbid and coexisting— Jennifer A. Namazy, Michael Schatz, and Sandra Gonzalez-Diaz -- Psychological factors comorbid and coexisting— Fulvio Braido, Tatiana Slavyanskaya, Giorgio Walter Canonica, Ilaria Baiardini, and Sepiashvili Revaz -- Asthma, substance abuse, and tobacco use— Riccardo Polosa and Pasquale Caponnetto -- Exercise-induced bronchoconstriction and asthma— Matteo Bonini, André Moreira, and Sergio Bonini -- Environmental risk factors in asthma— Tari Haahtela and Ömer Kalayci -- Age and asthma— Chelle Pope, Richard deShazo, and James King -- Atopic dermatitis, food allergy, and anaphylaxis comorbid and coexisting— Scott Sicherer, Hugh A. Sampson, Julie Wang, and Alessandro Fiocchi. Subjects: Asthma--complications. Asthma--diagnosis. Diagnosis, Differential. Respiratory Tract Diseases--complications. Respiratory Tract Diseases--diagnosis. Notes: "A World Federation of Allergy, Asthma & Clinical Immunology Societies." Includes bibliographical references and index.

Beyond the NICU: comprehensive care of the high-risk infant LCCN: 2014013204 Main title: Beyond the NICU: comprehensive care of the high-risk infant— edited by William F. Malcolm, MD, Associate Professor of Pediatrics, Director, Intermediate Level Nurseries, Division of Neonatal-Perinatal Medicine, Duke University Medical Center, Durham, North Carolina; consultants, Ricki F. Goldstein, MD, Professor of Pediatrics, Director, High-Risk Infant Follow-Up Program, Division of Neonatal-Perinatal Medicine, Duke University Medical Center, durham, North Carolina, Richard J. Martin, MD, Drusinsky-Fanaroff Chair in Neonatology, Professor of Pediatrics, Rainbow Babies & Children's Hospital, Case Western Reserve University, Cleveland, Ohio, Betty Vohr, MD, Professor of Pediatrics, Medical Director, Neonatal Follow-Up Program, Women & Infants Hospital, Alpert Medical School of Brown University, Providence, Rhode Island. Published/Produced: New York: McGraw-Hill Education, [2015] ©2015 Description: xxiv, 968 pages: illustrations (some color); 22 cm ISBN: 9780071748582 (paperback: alk. paper) 007174858X (paperback: alk. paper) LC classification: RJ254 .B49 2015 Variant title: Beyond the neonatal intensive care unit Related names: Malcolm, William F. (William Ferris),

1969- editor. Summary: "Beyond the NICU: Comprehensive Care of the High-Risk Infant delivers practical, evidence-based strategies for the care of convalescing NICU graduates in both inpatient and outpatient settings. In four sections, the book covers common problems shared by high-risk infants, role of various care providers from parents to specialists and timely interventions of therapy, timing and execution of transitioning the infant from intensive to convalescent care and from hospital to home, the etiology of chronic conditions affecting high-risk infants, details of convalescent care, discharge planning, and follow-up care for pediatricians"-- Provided by publisher. Contents: Machine generated contents note: Section 1 Introduction -- 1 History of the NICU -- 2 Commonalities of High Risk Infants: They're not all Preemies -- 3 Provider roles -- 4 Parent roles/wishes -- 5 Transitions for the High Risk Infant -- 6 Essential Components of a Comprehensive Follow-up Clinic -- Section 2 Medical Care of the Preterm Infant -- 7 Respiratory conditions of the preterm infant -- 8 Apnea and bradycardia -- 9 Patent ductus arteriosus -- 10 Adrenal Insufficiency -- 11 Nutrition and growth -- 12 Breastfeeding in the NICU Graduate -- 13 Necrotizing enterocolitis and short bowel syndrome -- 14 Gastroesophageal reflux -- 15 Catch-up Growth and Failure to thrive -- 16 Hypertension in the NICU Graduate -- 17 Anemia of prematurity -- 18 Thrombosis and Hematological Issues in the NICU Graduate -- 19 Hyperbilirubinemia -- 20 Endocrinopathies of the Preterm Infant -- 21 Bone Health -- 22 IVH, PVL, hypdrocephalus -- 23 Retinopathy of prematurity and ophthalmologic issues -- 24 Cerebral Palsy -- 25 Autism Spectrum Disorder -- 26 Intrauterine growth restriction -- 27 Post-NICU Issues of Multiple Gestation -- 28 Late Preterm Infants -- 29 Surgical issues -- Section 3 Medical Care of the Term Infant -- 30 Pulmonary Hypertension -- 31 Congenital diaphragmatic hernia -- 32 Congenital heart disease -- 33 ECMO and post-ECMO care -- 34 Congenital Intestinal anomalies -- 35 Maternal and neonatal infections -- 36 Birth asphyxia and HIE -- 37 Neonatal abstinence syndrome -- 38 Neural tube defects -- 39 Neonatal seizures and Infantile spasms -- 40 Infant of a diabetic mother -- 41 Down Syndrome --

Section 4 Developmental Care of the High Risk Infant -- 42 Early developmental issues in the NICU -- 43 NICU environment -- 44 Gross motor development -- 45 Fine motor development -- 46 Speech and language development -- 47 Feeding Issues in the NICU Graduate -- 48 Hearing Loss -- 49 Neurodevelopmental testing -- 50 Neurodevelopmental outcomes -- 51 Family centered care and social issues -- 52 Palliative care -- 53 Early Intervention Services -- 54 Resources for providers and parents -- Appendices -- App A Discharging the high-risk infant -- App B Equipment needs of the high risk infant -- App C Medications -- App D Tests/Procedures -- App E Telephone Triage -- App F Coding and Billing. Subjects: Infant, Premature, Diseases--therapy. Infant, Premature. Comprehensive Health Care. Infant, Newborn, Diseases--therapy. Intensive Care, Neonatal. Notes: Includes bibliographical references and index.

Clinical handbook of pediatric gastroenterology LCCN: 2014037654 Main title: Clinical handbook of pediatric gastroenterology— edited by Rosemary J. Pauley-Hunter, Lisa Philichi. Edition: Second edition. Published/Produced: [Omaha]: The Association of Pediatric Gastroenterology and Nutrition Nurses, 2015. Description: p.; cm. ISBN: 9781576264850 (pbk.: alk. paper) LC classification: RJ446 Related names: Pauley-Hunter, Rosemary J., editor. Philichi, Lisa., editor. Association of Pediatric Gastroenterology and Nutrition Nurses. Contents: Abdominal pain— Rosemary J. Pauley-Hunter, Daphne Pierce-Smith, and Robin Shannon -- Allergic Conditions of the Gastrointestinal Tract— Rosemary J. Pauley-Hunter -- Celiac Disease— Mary-Alice M. Tully -- Constipation and Encopresis— Lisa Philichi -- Cyclic Vomiting Syndrome— Adelina Ferraro McDuffie and Anne Wuerth -- Diarrhea— Patricia A. Bierly -- Failure to Thrive— Kimberly S. Jarczyk, Shari Huffman, and Kelli Bissell -- Gastroesophageal Reflux— Lisa Philichi -- Gastrointestinal Bleeding— Robin Shannon -- The A, B, and C of Hepatitis— Patricia Turner -- Inflammatory Bowel Disease— Susan N. Peck -- Liver Disease— Angela Tendick, Cheryl Calabro, and Kristin Peterson-Madden -- Obesity— Kathleen Milliken and Nancy Murray -- Pancreatitis— Elizabeth Goldberg and Clare Ceballos -- Short Bowel Syndrome— Rosemary J. Pauley-Hunter, Rebecca C. Ratcliff, and Elizabeth E. Gleghorn -- GI Transplant— Cindy R. Brown, Shari Huffman, Brandi Gerhardt, and Patricia Turner -- Diagnostic Studies— Diane Kocovsky -- GI Medications— Kathleen M. Gura, Shari Huffman, Lisa Philichi, and Maureen Egan -- Nutrition— Laura E. Beerman -- Feeding Tubes— Karen Sherry, Lillian R. Sablan, Corrine L. Maurins, and Emmala Ryan Shonce -- Growth Charts and Body Composition Analysis— Kimberly S. Jarczyk. Subjects: Gastrointestinal Diseases. Child. Infant. Liver Diseases. Pancreatic Diseases. Notes: Includes bibliographical references and index.

Diagnosis and treatment of gastroesophageal reflux disease. LCCN: 2015944713 Main title: Diagnosis and treatment of gastroesophageal reflux disease. Published/Produced: New York, NY: Springer Berlin Heidelberg, 2015. Description: pages cm

Everything guide to the acid reflux diet LCCN: 2014046373 Personal name: Rosick, Edward R. Main title: Everything guide to the acid reflux diet— Edward R. Rosick, DO, MPH, DABIHM. Published/Produced: Avon, Massachusetts: Adams Media, 2015. Description: pages cm ISBN: 9781440586262 (pb) 1440586268 (pb) LC classification: RC815.7 .R598 2015 Subjects: Gastroesophageal reflux--Popular works. Gastroesophageal reflux--Diet therapy. Gastroesophageal reflux--Diet therapy--Recipes. Notes: Includes bibliographical references and index.

Gastroesophageal reflux and the lung LCCN: 2012951839 Personal name: Meyer, Keith C. Main title: Gastroesophageal reflux and the lung— Keith C. Meyer, Ganesh Raghu, editors. Published/Produced: New York: Humana Press, [2013] Description: xii, 275 pages: illustrations (some color); 24 cm ISBN: 9781461455011 (hdbk.: acid-free paper) LC classification: RC815.7 .M49 2013 Related names: Raghu, Ganesh. Subjects: Gastroesophageal reflux. Lungs--Diseases.

Handbook of gastrointestinal motility and functional disorders LCCN: 2015004809 Main title:

Handbook of gastrointestinal motility and functional disorders— edited by Satish S.C. Rao, MD, PhD, FRCP, Professor of Medicine, Chief, Gastroenterology/Hepatology, Director, Digestive Health Center, Medical College of Georgia, Georgia Regents University, Henry P. Parkman, MD, Professor of Medicine, Head of GI Motility Laboratory, Gastrointestinal Section, Department of Medicine, Temple University Hospital, Richard W. McCallum, MD, FACP, FRACP (AUST), FAGG, AGAF, Professor of Medicine and Founding Chair, Department of Internal Medicine, Director, Center for Neurogastroenterology and GI Motility, Texas Tech University Health Sciences Center, Paul L. Foster School of Medicine. Published/Produced: Thorofare, NJ: SLACK Incorporated, [2015] ©2015 Description: xviii, 348 pages: illustrations (chiefly color); 26 cm ISBN: 9781617118180 (alk. paper) 1617118184 (alk. paper) LC classification: RC811 .H36 2015 RC802 Related names: Rao, Satish S. C., editor. Parkman, Henry P., editor. McCallum, Richard W., editor. Contents: Esophageal symptoms: dysphagia, heartburn, and esophageal chest pain -- Gastroesophageal reflux disease -- Achalasia -- Esophageal spasm, hypercontractile, and hypertensive motility disorders -- Cricopharyngeal disorders -- Esophageal hypersensitivity -- Nausea and vomiting, abdominal pain, postprandial fullness, and early satiety -- Gastroparesis -- Functional dyspepsia -- Dumping syndrome -- Cyclic vomiting syndrome -- Rumination syndrome -- Small intestinal motility symptoms: bloating, distension, and gas -- Chronic intestinal pseudoobstruction -- Small intestinal bacterial overgrowth -- Food intolerance and dietary concepts in functional bowel disorders -- Colonic symptoms: constipation, diarrhea, and fecal incontinence -- Irritable bowel syndrome -- Slow transit constipation -- Dyssynergic defecation and constipation -- Fecal incontinence -- Anorectal disorders: fecal impaction, descending perineum syndrome, rectocele, and levator ani syndrome -- Diabetes and the gut -- Scleroderma and the gut -- Opiate-induced bowel dysfunction. Subjects: Gastrointestinal system--Motility--Disorders--Handbooks. Gastrointestinal system--Diseases--Handbooks.

Gastrointestinal Diseases--Handbooks. Gastrointestinal Motility--Handbooks. Notes: Includes bibliographical references.

Low acid slow cooking: over 100 reflux-free recipes for the electric slow cooker LCCN: 2014395673 Personal name: DeVito, Dominique, author. Main title: Low acid slow cooking: over 100 reflux-free recipes for the electric slow cooker— Dominique DeVito; with Breea Johnson. Edition: 1st ed. Published/Produced: Kennebunkport, Maine: Cider Mill Press, [2013] ©2013 Description: 255 pages color illustrations; 23 cm ISBN: 9781604333176 (paperback) 1604333170 (paperback) Related names: Johnson, Breea, author. Contents: Introduction: Eating to manage acid reflux -- Slow going: a guide to slow cooking and the wonders of slow cooking -- Low-acid breakfasts -- Soups that don't simmer your insides -- Pasta sauces: no tomatoes allowed! -- Poultry is your low-acid friend -- Fish dishes that fulfill wishes -- Veggies to tantalize yet minimize -- Side dishes that won't bubble over -- Dessert without hurt. Subjects: Gastroesophageal reflux--Diet therapy--Recipes. Electric cooking, Slow. Notes: Includes index.

Practical manual of gastroesophageal reflux disease LCCN: 2012030222 Main title: Practical manual of gastroesophageal reflux disease— edited by Marcelo F. Vela, Joel E. Richter, John E. Pandolfino. Published/Created: Chichester, West Sussex, UK; Hoboken, NJ: Wiley-Blackwell, 2013. Description: x, 342 p.: ill. (some col.); 25 cm. ISBN: 9780470656266 (pbk.: alk. paper) 9781118444788 (obook) 9781118444795 (mobi) 9781118444801 (epub) 9781118444825 (ebook/epdf) LC classification: RC815.7 .P733 2013 Related names: Vela, Marcelo F. Richter, Joel E. Pandolfino, John E. Subjects: Gastroesophageal reflux--Handbooks, manuals, etc. Notes: Includes bibliographical references and index.

Principles of deglutition: a multidisciplinary text for swallowing and its disorders LCCN: 2012943384 Main title: Principles of deglutition: a multidisciplinary text for swallowing and its disorders— Reza Shaker ... [et al.], editors. Published/Created: New York:

Springer, c2013. Description: xix, 1017 p.: ill. (some col.); 27 cm. ISBN: 9781461437932 (alk. paper) 1461437938 (alk. paper) LC classification: RC815.2 .P75 2013 Related names: Shaker, Reza. Partial contents: General Aspects of Deglutition. Overview of Deglutition and Digestion; Gustation, Olfaction and Deglutition; Coordination of Deglutition and Respiration; Airway Protective Mechanisms, Reciprocal Physiology of the Deglutitive Axis -- Central Control of Deglutition. Cerebral Cortical Control of Deglutition; Brainstem Control of Deglutition: Swallowing Pattern Generator; Brainstem Control of Deglutition: Brainstem Neural Circuits and Mediators Regulating Swallowing -- Preparatory/Oral Phase of Deglutition. Oral Phase Preparation and Propulsion: Anatomy, Physiology, Rheology, Mastication and Transport; Deglutitive Oral Pressure Phenomena; Effect of Aging on the Oral Phase of Deglutition; Nascent Oral Phase -- Pharyngeal Phase of Deglutition. Development, Anatomy and Physiology of the Pharynx; Development, Anatomy and Physiology of the Larynx; Development, Anatomy and Physiology of the Lungs; Effect of Aging of the Pharynx and the UES; Nascent Pharynx, Physiology, Reflexes -- UES and its Deglutitive Function. Development, Anatomy and Physiology of the Upper Esophageal Sphincter and Pharyngo-Esophageal Junction; Deglutitive Pharyngeal and UES Pressure Phenomena -- Esophageal Phase of Deglutition. Development, Anatomy and Physiology of the Esophagus; Normal Aging and the Esophagus; Nascent Esophagus, Sensory-Motor Physiology during Maturation -- Esophageal Motility and Its Deglutitive Function. Esophageal Motor Physiology; Sphincter Mechanisms at the Esophago-Gastric Junction; Motility and Pressure Phenomena of the Esophagus -- Oral/Pharyngeal Phase Dysphagia. Symptom Indices for Dysphagia Assessment and Management; Cerebro-Vascular Accidents and Dysphagia; Progressive Neurologic Disease and Dysphagia (including Parkinson's Disease, Multiple Sclerosis, Amyotrophic Lateral Sclerosis, Myasthenia Gravis, Post Polio Syndrome); Disorders of Appetite, Eating and Swallowing in the Dementias; Dystrophies and Myopathies (including Muscular,

Oculopharyngeal); Dysphagia Secondary to the Effects of Chemo and Radiation Therapy; Swallowing Syncope; Globus Pharyngeus; Deglutition in Patients with Tracheostomy, Nasogastric Tubes and Orogastric Tubes; Dysphagia Secondary to Systemic Diseases -- Upper Esophageal Sphincter Opening Dysfunction. Zenker's Diverticulum; Cricopharyngeal Bar; Cricopharyngeal Achalasia; UES Opening Muscle Dysfunction -- Esophageal Phase Dysphagia: Motor Disorders. Achalasia and Ineffective Esophageal Motility; Esophageal Spasm/Non-Cardiac Chest Pain Hypertensive Esophageal Peristalsis (Nutcracker Esophagus) Hypertensive Lower Esophageal Sphincter -- Esophageal Phase Dysphagia: Structural Abnormalities. Benign and Malignant Tumors of the Esophagus; Strictures, Rings, Webs (peptic, caustic, radiation, anastomotic); Esophageal Foreign Bodies: Food Impaction and Foreign Bodies; Post-Surgical Dysphagia: Post-Nissen Fundoplication, C-spine surgery, Thyroid surgery, Gastric Banding, Gastric Bypass; Drug-induced Esophageal Injury; Infectious Esophagitis; Eosinophilic Esophagitis; Gastroesophageal Reflux Disease; Barrett's Esophagus; Extraesophageal Manifestations of Reflux Disease and Dysphagia; Hiatal Hernia -- Eating Disorders. Psychogenic Dysphagia; Rumination Syndrome -- Treatment Options for Deglutition Disorders. Compensatory Management and Treatment in Dysphagia; Rehabilitative Treatments; Electrical Stimulation Treatment; Pharmacotherapy of UES Spastic Disorder; Open and Endoscopic Cricopharyngeal Myotomy; Surgical Treatment of Zenker's Diverticulum; Dilatations (UES, Esophagus, LES) Balloon Dilations, Bougies; Esophageal Stenting for Relief of Dysphagia; Botulinum Toxin for LES Spastic Disorders; Surgical Treatment of Achalasia and Spastic Esophageal Disorders; Vocal Fold Medialization, Arytenoid Adduction, and Partial Pharyngectomy; Laryngohyoid Suspension; Surgical Management of Life-Threatening Aspiration; Anti-Reflux Surgery; Tube Feeding: Indications, Considerations and Technique. Subjects: Deglutition disorders. Deglutition. Deglutition Disorders--therapy. Deglutition--physiology. Deglutition Disorders--

physiopathology. Notes: Includes bibliographical references and index.

Proton pump inhibitors: a balanced view LCCN: 2013020683 Uniform title: Proton pump inhibitors (2013) Main title: Proton pump inhibitors: a balanced view— volume editors, Tsutomu Chiba, Kyoto, Peter Malfertheiner, Magdeburg, Hiroshi Satoh, Kyoto. Published/Produced: Basel; New York: Karger, 2013. Description: vii, 119 pages: illustrations (some color); 26 cm. ISBN: 9783318024159 (hard cover: alk. paper) LC classification: RC827 .P76 2013 Related names: Chiba, Tsutomu, editor of compilation. Malfertheiner, P. (Peter), 1950- editor of compilation. Satoh, Hiroshi, editor of compilation. Subjects: Peptic Ulcer--drug therapy. Gastroesophageal Reflux--drug therapy. Proton Pump Inhibitors--pharmacology. Proton Pump Inhibitors--therapeutic use. Risk Assessment. Notes: Includes bibliographical references and indexes. Series: Frontiers of gastrointestinal research, 0302-0665; vol. 32 Frontiers of gastrointestinal research; v. 32. 0302-0665

Reflux laryngitis and related disorders LCCN: 2013011269 Personal name: Sataloff, Robert Thayer, author. Main title: Reflux laryngitis and related disorders— Robert T. Sataloff, Philip Katz, Mary J. Hawkshaw, Dahlia Sataloff. Edition: Fourth edition Published/Produced: San Diego: Plural Publishing, [2013] ©2013 Description: xiv, 227 pages: illustrations; 24 cm ISBN: 9781597565387 (alk. paper) 1597565385 (alk. paper) LC classification: RF520 .R44 2013 Related names: Katz, Philip O., 1953- author. Hawkshaw, Mary, author. Sataloff, Dahlia, author. Contents: Anatomy and physiology of the voice -- Anatomy and physiology of the esophagus and its sphincters -- New concepts in the anatomy and physiology of the anti-reflux barrier— Larry Miller, Kian Makipour, Pathikonda Murali, Anil Vegesna -- Gastroesophageal reflux disease: an overview of clinical presentation and epidemiology -- Reflux laryngitis and other otolaryngologic manifestations of laryngopharyngeal reflux -- Diagnostic tests for gastroesophageal reflux -- Behavioral and medical management of gastroesophageal reflux disease -

- Surgical therapy for gastroesophageal reflux disease. Subjects: Laryngitis--diagnosis. Laryngitis--etiology. Laryngopharyngeal Reflux--complications. Laryngopharyngeal Reflux--therapy. Notes: Includes bibliographical references and index.

Sabiston textbook of surgery: the biological basis of modern surgical practice. LCCN: 2011040621 Main title: Sabiston textbook of surgery: the biological basis of modern surgical practice. Edition: 19th ed.— [edited by] Courtney M. Townsend Jr. ... [et al.]. Published/Created: Philadelphia, PA: Elsevier Saunders, c2012. Description: xxv, 2124 p.: ill. (some col.); 29 cm. ISBN: 9781437715606 (hardcover: alk. paper) 1437715605 (hardcover: alk. paper) 9781455711468 (international ed.) 1455711462 (international ed.) LC classification: RD31 .T473 2012 Variant title: Textbook of surgery Related names: Sabiston, David C., 1924-2009. Townsend, Courtney M. Summary: "Sabiston Textbook of Surgery is your ultimate foundation for confident surgical decision making. Covering the very latest science and data affecting your treatment planning, this esteemed medical reference helps you make the most informed choices so you can ensure the best outcome for every patient."-- Publisher's website. Contents: History of surgery -- Ethics and professionalism in surgery -- Molecular and cell biology -- The inflammatory response -- Shock, electrolytes, and fluid -- Metabolism in surgical patients -- Wound healing -- Regenerative medicine -- Evidence-based surgery: critically assessing surgical literature -- Perioperative patient safety -- Principles of preoperative and operative surgery -- Surgical infections and antibiotic use -- Surgical complications -- Surgery in the geriatric patient -- Morbid obesity -- Anesthesiology principles, pain management, and conscious sedation -- Emerging technology in surgery: informatics, robotics, and electronics -- Management of acute trauma -- The difficult abdominal wall -- Emergency care of musculoskeletal injuries -- Burns -- Bites and stings -- Surgical critical care -- Bedside surgical procedures -- The surgeon's role in mass casualty incidents -- Transplantation immunobiology and immunosuppression -- Liver transplantation -- Kidney and pancreas transplantation -- Small bowel transplantation -- Tumor biology and tumor markers -- Tumor immunology and immunotherapy -- Melanoma and cutaneous malignancies -- Soft tissue sarcomas -- Bone tumors -- Head and neck -- Diseases of the breast -- Breast reconstruction -- Thyroid -- The parathyroid glands -- Endocrine pancreas -- The adrenal glands -- The multiple endocrine neoplasia syndromes -- Esophagus -- Hiatal hernia and gastroesophageal reflux disease -- Abdominal wall, umbilicus, peritoneum, mesenteries, omentum, and retroperitoneum -- Hernias -- Acute abdomen -- Acute gastrointestinal hemorrhage -- Stomach -- Small intestine -- The appendix -- Colon and rectum -- Anus -- The liver -- Biliary system -- Exocrine pancreas -- The spleen -- Lung, chest wall, pleura, and mediastinum -- Congenital heart disease -- Acquired heart disease: coronary insufficiency -- Acquired heart disease: valvular -- Aorta -- Peripheral arterial occlusive disease -- Vascular trauma -- Venous disease -- The lymphatics -- Pediatric surgery -- Neurosurgery -- Plastic surgery -- Hand surgery -- Gynecologic surgery -- Surgery in the pregnant patient -- Urologic surgery. Subjects: Surgery--Textbooks. Surgical Procedures, Operative. General Surgery. Perioperative Care. Notes: Includes bibliographical references and index.

The 5-minute pediatric consult
LCCN: 2012012664 Main title: The 5-minute pediatric consult— editor, M. William Schwartz; associate editors, Louis M. Bell, Jr. ... [et al.]; assistant editor, Charles I. Schwartz. Edition: 6th ed. Published/Created: Philadelphia: Wolters Kluwer/Lippincott Williams & Wilkins, c2012. Description: xxx, 1113 p.: ill.; 28 cm. ISBN: 9781451116564 (hardback: alk. paper) 145111656X (hardback: alk. paper) LC classification: RJ48 .A15 2012 Variant title: Five-minute pediatric consult Related names: Schwartz, M. William, 1935- Summary: "The 5 Minute Pediatric Consult provides immediate, practical advice on problems seen in infants, children, and adolescents. More than 450 diseases and conditions are covered in the fast-access two-page outline format that makes The 5-Minute Consult Series titles so popular among busy clinicians. Other features

include a Chief Complaints section addressing the workup and treatment of 50 signs and symptoms, plus a medication index, syndromes glossary, surgical glossary, laboratory values, and tables all for quick reference saving you time and helping to treat your patients more efficiently.In this sixth edition, the 5 Minute Pediatric Consult also offers free 30 day access to the 5minuteconsult Pediatric website -- a clinical decision support tool -- that can be accessed by the health care providers to address questions on-the-go via website or mobile.New Features: New topics for this edition include: Amenorrhea, Asberger Syndrome, Dental Trauma, Head banging, Mental Retardation, Narcolepsy, Obsessive Compulsive Disorder, Separation Anxiety and Social Anxiety Free 30 Day Access to the 5minuteconsult Pediatric Website Includes More than 450 diseases and conditions to support your patient care decisions Patient education handouts from AAP to help educate your patients Hundreds of Images from Chung's "Visual Diagnosis and Treatment in Pediatrics" and other reputable sources to provide you with quick visual guidance Immunization schedules and charts at your fingertips to save you time from searching Content is optimized for handheld devices so you have access to the content anytime, anywhere Updates to content made on a regular basis to keep you abreast of the latest content Visit 5minuteconsult.com and click on the "go to pediatric consult tab" to learn more about your free access and begin using today!"-- Provided by publisher. Contents: Abdominal Mass -- Abdominal migraine -- Abdominal pain -- Abnormal bleeding -- Acetaminophen poisoning -- Acne -- Acquired hypothyroidism -- Acute drug withdrawal -- Acute kidney injury -- Acute lymphoblastic leukemia -- Acute myeloid leukemia -- Adenovirus infection -- Alcohol (ethanol) intoxication -- Allergic child -- Alopecia (hair loss) -- Alpha-1-Antitrypsin defficiency -- Altitude illness -- Amblyopia -- Amebiasis -- Amenorrhea -- Anearobic infections -- Anaphylaxis -- Anemia of chronic disease (Anemia of inflammation) -- Anicryptococcal infections -- Ankylosing spondylitis -- Anomalous coronary artery -- Anorexia nervosa -- Anthrax -- Aplastic anemia -- Appendicitis

- Dermatomyositis/ Polymyositis -- Developmental disabilities -- Developmental dysplasia of the hip -- Diabetes insipidus -- Diabetes mellitus -- Diabetic ketoacidosis -- Diaper rash -- Diaphragmatic hernia (Congenital) -- Diarrhea -- Diphtheria -- Diskitis -- Disorders of sex development -- Disseminated intravascular coagulation -- Down (Trisomy 21) Syndrome -- Drowning -- Dysfunctional uterine bleeding -- Dysmenorrhea -- Dyspnea -- Dysuria -- Earache -- Edema -- Ehrlichiosis and anaplasmosis -- Encephalitis -- Encopresis -- Endocarditis -- Enuresis -- Endocarditis -- Epiglottitis -- Epstein Barr virus (Infectious Mononucleosis -- Erythema multiforme -- Erythema Nodosum -- Ewing Sarcoma -- Exstrophy of the bladder, cloacal exstrophy, and epispadias -- Failure to thrive -- Feeding disorders -- Fetal alcohol syndrome -- Fever and petechiae -- Fever of unknown cause -- Floppy infant syndrome -- Food allergy -- Food poisoning or foodborne illness -- Fragile X syndrome -- Frostbite -- Functional diarrhea of infancy or toddLer's diarrhea -- Fungal skin infections (Dermatophyte infections, Candidiasis, and Tinea Versicolor) -- Gastritis -- Gastroesophageal reflux -- German measles (third disease, Rubella) -- Giardiasis -- Gingivitis -- Glaucoma--congenital -- Glomerulonephritis -- Gluecose-6-phosphate dehydrogenase deficiency -- Goiter -- Gonococcal infections -- Graft versus host disease -- Graves disease -- Growth hormone deficiency -- Guillain-Barre syndrome -- Gynecomastia -- Hand, foot, and mouth disease -- Hantavirus -- Head banging -- Headache and migraine -- Heat stroke and related illness -- Hemangiomas and other vascular lesions -- Hematuria -- Hemolysis -- Hemolysis -- Hemolytic disease of the newborn -- Hemolytic uremic syndrome -- Hemophilia -- Hemoptysis -- Henoch-Schonlein purpura -- Hepatic failure -- Hepatomegaly -- Hereditary Angioedema -- Hereditary spherocytosis -- Heroin intoxication -- Herpes simplex virus -- Hiccups -- Hirschsprung disease -- Histiocytosis -- Histoplasmosis -- Hodgkin Lymphoma -- Human immunodeficiency virus infection -- Human papilloma virus -- Hydrocephalus -- Hydronephrosis -- Hyperimmunoglobulinemia E Syndrome -- Hyperinsulinism -- Hyperlipidemia -- Hypertention

-- Hypogammaglobulinemia -- Hypoparathyroidism -- Hypoplastic left heart syndrome -- Hypospadias -- Idiopathic intracranial hypertension (Pseudotumor cerebri) -- Idiopathic Thrombocytopenic purpura -- Immune deficiency -- Immunoglobulin a deficiency -- Imperforate anus -- Impetigo -- In Inappropriate antidiuretic hormone secretion -- Infantile spasms -- Influenza -- Inguinal hernia -- Intestinal obstruction -- Intoeing-tibial torsion -- Intracranial hemorrhage -- Intussusception -- Iron deficiency anemia -- Iron poisoning -- Irritable bowel syndrome -- Jaundice -- Kawasaki disease -- Knee pain, Anterior/Patellofemoral malalignment syndrome -- Lacrimal duct obstruction -- Lactos intolerance -- Lead poisoning -- Learning disabilities -- Luekocytosis -- Lice (Pediculosis) -- Lower GI bleeding -- Lupus erythematosus -- Lyme disease -- Lymphadenopathy -- Malabsorption -- Malaria -- Mammalian bites -- Mastoiditis -- Measles (Rubeola, first disease) -- Meckel diverticulum -- Mediastinal mass -- Megaloblastic anemia -- Meningitis -- Meningococcemia -- Mental retardation -- Mesenteric adenitis -- Metabolic diseases in hypoglycemic newborns -- Metabolic diseases in acidotic newborns -- Metabolic diseases in Hyperammonemic newborns -- Metabolic syndrome -- Methemoglobinemia -- Microcytic anemia -- Milia -- Milk protein intolerance -- Mumps/Parotitis -- Munchausen syndrome by proxy -- Muscular dystrophies -- Myasthenia gravis -- Myocarditis -- Narcolepsy -- Neck masses -- Necrotizing entercolitis -- Neonatal alloimmune thrombocytopenia -- Neonatal apnea -- Neonatal cholestasis -- Nephrotic syndrome -- Neural tube defects -- Neuroblastoma -- Neurofibromatosis -- Neutropenia -- Non-Hodgkin Lymphoma -- Nosebleeds (Epistaxis) -- Obesity -- Obsessive compulsive disorder -- Obstetric brachial plexus (ERB) palsy -- Omphalitis -- Osteogenesis imperfecta -- Osteosarcoma -- Osteomyelitis -- Otitis externa -- Otitis media -- Pallor -- Pancreatic Pseudocyst -- Pancreatitis -- Panhypopituitarism -- Parvovirus B 19 (Erythema Infectiosum, fifth disease) -- Patent ductus arteriosus -- Pelvic inflammatory disease (PID) -- Penile and foreskin problems --

Pericarditis -- Periodic breathing -- Periorbital cellulitis -- Perirectal abscess -- Peritonitis -- Peritonsillar abscess -- Persistent Pulmonary Hypertension of the newborn (PPHN) -- Perthes disease -- Pertussis -- Pharyngitis -- Photosensitivity -- Pinworms -- Plague -- Pleural effusion -- Pneumoystic Jiroveci (Previously known as Pneumocystic Carnii Pneumonis) -- Pneumonia--Bacterial -- Pneumothorax -- Polyarteritis Nodosa -- Polycystic kidney disease -- Polycystic ovary syndrome -- Polycythemia -- Polyps, intestinal -- Porencephaly cortical dysplasia/neuronal migration disorders-malformations of cortical development -- Portal hypertension -- Posterior urethral valve -- Premature adrenarche -- Premature thelarche -- Premenstrual syndrome (PMS) -- Primary adrenal insufficiency -- Prion diseases (Transmissible spongiform encephalophathies) -- Probiotics -- Prolonged QT interval syndrome -- Protein-Energy malnutrition (Kwashiorkor) -- Proteinuria -- Prune belly syndrome -- Pruritus -- Psittacosis -- Psoriasis -- Pubertal delay -- Pulmonary embolism -- Pulmonary hypertension -- Purpura fulminans -- Pyelonephritis -- Pyloric stenosis -- Rabies -- Rectal prolapse -- Refractive error -- Renal artery stenosis -- Renal tubular acidosis -- Renal venous thrombosis -- Respiratory syncytial virus (RSV) -- Retinoblastoma -- Retropharyngeal abscess -- Reye Syndrome -- Rhabdomyolysis -- Rhabdomyosarcoma -- Rheumatic fever -- Rhinitis, Allergic -- Rickets -- Rickettsial disease -- Rocky Mountain Spotted Fever -- Roseola -- Rotavirus -- Salicylate poisoning (Aspirin) -- Salmonella infections -- Sarcoidosis -- Scabies -- Scarlet fever -- Scleroderma -- Scoliosis (Idiopathic) -- Seborrheic dermatitis -- Seizures-febrile -- Seizures, partial and generalized -- Separation anxiety disorder -- Sepsis -- Septic arthritis -- Serum Sickness -- Severe acute respiratory syndrome (SARS) -- Severe combined immunodeficiency -- Sexual abuse -- Sexual ambiguity -- Sexual precocity -- Short-bowel syndrome -- Short stature -- Sickle cell disease -- Sinusitis -- Sleep apnea--obstructive sleep apnea syndrome -- Slipped capital femoral epiphysis -- Smallpox (Variola virus) --

Snake and insect bites -- Social anxiety disorder -- Sore throat -- Speech delay -- Speech problems -- Spinal muscular atrophy -- Splenomegaly -- Staphylococcal scaled skin syndrome (SSSS) -- Status epilepticus -- Stevens-Johnson syndrome and toxic epidermal necrolysis -- Stomatitis -- Strabismus -- Strep infection: invasive Group A Ç-hemolytic streptococcus -- Stroke -- Stuttering -- Subdural hematoma -- Substance use disorders -- Sudden Infant Death Syndrome (SIDS) -- Suicide -- Superior Mesenteric Artery syndrome -- Superior Mesenteric artery syndrome -- Supraventricular tachycardia -- Sympathomimetic poisoning -- Syncope -- Synovitis--transient -- Syphilis -- Tapeworm -- Teething -- Tendonitis -- Teratoma -- Tenanus -- Tetralogy of Fallot -- Thalassemia -- Thoracic insufficiency syndrome -- Thrombosis -- Tick fever -- Tics -- Toxic alcohols -- Toxic Shock syndrome -- Toxoplasmosis -- Tracheitis -- Tracheoesophageal fistula and esophageal atresia -- Tracheomalacia/laryngomalacia -- Transfusion reaction -- Transient erythroblastopenia of childhood -- Transient Trachypnea of the Newborn (TTN) -- Transposition of the great arteries -- Transverse myelitis -- Trichinosis -- Tuberculosis -- Tuberous sclerosis complex -- Tularemia -- Ulcerative colitis -- Upper gastrointestional bleeding -- Ureteropelvic junction obstruction -- Urethral prolapse -- Urinary tract infection -- Urticaria -- Vaccine adverse events -- Vaginitis -- Vascular brain lesions (Congenial) -- Ventricular septal defect -- Ventricular tachycardia -- Vesicoureteral reflux -- Viral hepatitis -- Volvulus -- Vomiting -- Von Willebrand disease -- Warts -- Weight loss -- West Nile Virus (And other Arbovirus Encephalitis) -- Wheezing -- Wilms tumor -- Wilson disease -- Wiskott-Aldrich syndrome -- Yersinia enterocolitica. Subjects: Pediatrics--Handbooks, manuals, etc. Pediatrics. Pediatrics--Handbooks. Notes: Includes bibliographical references and index. Series: 5-minute consult series 5-minute consult.

The acid reflux solution: a cookbook and lifestyle guide for healing heartburn naturally LCCN: 2011033896 Personal name: Rodriguez, Jorge E. Main title: The acid reflux solution: a cookbook and lifestyle guide for healing heartburn naturally— Jorge E. Rodriguez, Susan

Wyler. Edition: 1st ed. Published/Created: Berkeley: Ten Speed Press, 2012. Description: vii, 215 p.: col. ill.; 24 cm. ISBN: 9781607742272 (pbk.) 9781607742289 (ebook) LC classification: RC815.7 R59 2012 Related names: Wyler, Susan. Summary: "A full-color cookbook and health guide for heartburn sufferers that presents lifestyle recommendations, dietary guidelines, and 100 gourmet recipes to alleviate the symptoms of acid reflux. Millions of Americans suffer from acid reflux--and although medication can bring short-term relief, over time, drugs may have serious health consequences. In this combination cookbook and health guide, Dr. Jorge E. Rodriguez-- who suffers from acid reflux himself-- offers a simple plan for controlling reflux, including 100 delicious and reflux-free recipes that promote better health and weight loss. In fact, Dr. Rodriguez lost 35 pounds while writing (and following) the plan for this book. By busting popular myths and drawing on the latest evidence-based research, The Acid Reflux solution provides real heartburn relief even for longtime sufferers"-- Provided by publisher. "A combination health guide and cookbook that presents the latest evidence-based research, lifestyle recommendations, and dietary guidelines, along with 100 recipes to heal heartburn naturally"-- Provided by publisher. Subjects: Gastroesophageal reflux--Popular works. Gastroesophageal reflux--Diet therapy--Recipes. Cooking— Health & Healing— General Cooking— Health & Healing— Weight Control Health & Fitness— Diets Notes: Includes bibliographical references and index.

The complete idiot's guide to the acid reflux diet LCCN: 2011910192 Personal name: Bella, Maria A. Main title: The complete idiot's guide to the acid reflux diet— by Maria A. Bella. Published/Created: New York: Alpha Books, c2012. Description: xvii, 317 p.; 23 cm. ISBN: 9781615641406 (pbk.) 1615641408 (pbk.) LC classification: RC815.7 .B44 2012 Portion of title: Acid reflux diet Summary: Packed with tips for treating and relieving your acid reflux, this helpful guide give you everything you need to know to be free of acid reflux for good. Includes delicious recipes that won't aggravate your symptoms. Contents: A closer look at acid reflux -- Ensuring your success on the acid reflux diet -- Cooking and dining out strategies -- Recipes for reflux-free living. Subjects: Gastroesophageal reflux--Popular works. Heartburn--Popular works. Gastroesophageal reflux--Diet therapy. Heartburn--Diet therapy. Gastroesophageal reflux--Diet therapy--Recipes. Heartburn--Diet therapy--Recipes. Notes: Includes bibliographical references (p. [301]-302) and index. Series: Complete idiot's guide

What to feed your baby: cost-conscious nutrition for your infant LCCN: 2012047855 Personal name: Cohen, Stanley A., 1947- Main title: What to feed your baby: cost-conscious nutrition for your infant— Stan Cohen. Published/Produced: Lanham, Maryland: Rowman & Littlefield Publishers, Inc., [2013] Description: x, 261 pages: illustrations; 23 cm ISBN: 9781442219205 (pbk.: alk. paper) LC classification: RJ206 .C64 2013 Contents: First decisions -- Back to the breast -- Breastfeeding is almost as simple as it looks -- If you choose to use a bottle -- Specialty formulas for babies with problems -- Gastroesophageal reflux -- Colic and fussiness -- Pooping problems: red, white, blue or possibly loose -- Are allergies everywhere? -- Underweight or undergrown -- The premature infant -- Overweight or just plain healthy -- Infant foods and how to introduce them -- Transitioning to the real stuff -- Essential nutrients -- Transitioning to toddlerhood. Subjects: Infants--Nutrition. Children--Nutrition. Notes: Includes bibliographical references and index.

Your nutrition solution to acid reflux: a meal-based plan to help manage acid reflux, heartburn, and other symptoms of GERD LCCN: 2014000408 Personal name: Tessmer, Kimberly A., author. Main title: Your nutrition solution to acid reflux: a meal-based plan to help manage acid reflux, heartburn, and other symptoms of GERD— Kimberly A. Tessmer, RDN, LD. Published/Produced: Pompton Plains, N.J.: New Page Books, a division of The Career Press, Inc., [2014] ©2014 Description: 224 pages: illustrations; 21 cm ISBN: 9781601633231 (pbk.) 1601633238 (pbk.) LC classification: RC815.7 .T47 2014 Subjects: Gastroesophageal reflux--

Nutritional aspects. Gastroesophageal reflux--Diet therapy--Recipes. Form/Genre: Cookbooks. Notes: "Includes shopping and menu planning guide"--Cover. Includes bibliographical references (pages 209-216) and index.

INDEX

A

B

C

D

H

I

J

K

L

M

N

O

P

Q

R

S

T